Pediatric Anterior Cruciate Ligament Injury: A Focus on Prevention and Treatment in the Young Athlete

Guest Editor

THEODORE J. GANLEY, MD

CLINICS IN
SPORTS MEDICINE

www.sportsmed.theclinics.com

Consulting Editor
MARK D. MILLER, MD

October 2011 • Volume 30 • Number 4

SAUNDERS an imprint of ELSEVIER, Inc.

W.B. SAUNDERS COMPANY
A Division of Elsevier Inc.

1600 John F. Kennedy Blvd. • Suite 1800 • Philadelphia, Pennsylvania 19103

http://www.theclinics.com

CLINICS IN SPORTS MEDICINE Volume 30, Number 4
October 2011 ISSN 0278-5919, ISBN-13: 978-1-4557-1154-3

Editor: Jessica McCool

Clinics in Sports Medicine (ISSN 0278-5919) is published quarterly by Elsevier Inc., 360 Park Avenue South, New York, NY 10010-1710. Months of issue are January, April, July, and October. Business and Editorial Offices: 1600 John F. Kennedy Blvd., Ste. 1800, Philadelphia, PA 19103-2899. Customer Service Office: 3251 Riverport Lane, Maryland Heights, MO 63043. Periodicals postage paid at New York, NY and additional mailing offices. Subscription prices are $297.00 per year (US individuals), $466.00 per year (US institutions), $147.00 per year (US students), $337.00 per year (Canadian individuals), $563.00 per year (Canadian institutions), $205.00 (Canadian students), $409.00 per year (foreign individuals), $563.00 per year (foreign institutions), and $205.00 per year (foreign students). Foreign air speed delivery is included in all *Clinics* subscription prices. All prices are subject to change without notice. **POSTMASTER:** Send address changes to *Clinics in Sports Medicine,* Elsevier Health Sciences Division, Subscription Customer Service, 3251 Riverport Lane, Maryland Heights, MO 63043. Customer Service (orders, claims, online, change of address): Elsevier Health Sciences Division, Subscription Customer Service, 3251 Riverport Lane, Maryland Heights, MO 63043. Tel: 1-800-654-2452 (U.S. and Canada); 314-447-8871 (outside U.S. and Canada). Fax: 314-447-8029. E-mail: journalscustomerservice-usa@elsevier.com (for print support); journalsonlinesupport-usa@elsevier.com (for online support).

Reprints. For copies of 100 or more of articles in this publication, please contact the Commercial Reprints Department, Elsevier Inc., 360 Park Avenue South, New York, NY 10010-1710. Tel.: 212-633-3812; Fax: 212-462-1935; E-mail: reprints@elsevier.com.

Clinics in Sports Medicine is covered in *MEDLINE/PubMed (Index Medicus) Current Contents/Clinical Medicine, Excerpta Medica,* and *ISI/Biomed.*

Printed and bound by CPI Group (UK) Ltd, Croydon, CR0 4YY

Transferred to Digital Print 2011

Contributors

CONSULTING EDITOR

MARK D. MILLER, MD
S. Ward Casscells Professor of Orthopaedic Surgery, University of Virginia, Charlottesville, Virginia; Team Physician, James Madison University, Harrisonburg, Virginia

GUEST EDITOR

THEODORE J. GANLEY, MD
Sports Medicine Director, Division of Orthopaedic Surgery; The Sports Medicine Performance Centers, The Children's Hospital of Philadelphia; Associate Professor of Orthopaedic Surgery, The University of Pennsylvania School of Medicine, Philadelphia, Pennsylvania

AUTHORS

CHAD AARONS, MD
Tuckahoe Orthopaedic Associates, Richmond, Virginia

JAY C. ALBRIGHT, MD
Arnold Palmer Hospital for Children, Orlando, Florida

ALLEN F. ANDERSON, MD
Director, Tennessee Orthopaedic Alliance/The Lipscomb Clinic, Nashville, Tennessee

CHRISTIAN N. ANDERSON, MD
Resident, Department of Orthopaedic Surgery, Vanderbilt University Medical Center, Nashville, Tennessee

JAMES R. ANDREWS, MD
Medical Director and Chairman, American Sports Medicine Institute, Birmingham, Alabama

STEPHEN K. AOKI, MD
University of Utah School of Medicine, Salt Lake City, Utah

NICHOLAS A. BECK, BS
Division of Orthopaedic Surgery, The Children's Hospital of Philadelphia, Philadelphia, Pennsylvania

JENSEN L. BRENT, CSCS
Division of Sports Medicine, Cincinnati Children's Hospital Medical Center, Cincinnati, Ohio

MICHAEL T. BUSCH, MD
Director of Sports Medicine, Children's Healthcare of Atlanta, Atlanta, Georgia

JAMES L. CAREY, MD, MPH
Assistant Professor of Orthopaedic Surgery, University of Pennsylvania; Director of the Penn Center for Advanced Cartilage Repair and Osteochondritis Dissecans Treatment, Philadelphia, Pennsylvania

CORDELIA W. CARTER, MD
Postgraduate Fellow, Division of Sports Medicine, Children's Hospital Boston, Boston, Massachusetts

ANNE MARIE CHICORELL, DO, MPH
Fellow, Division of Sports Medicine, Department of Orthopaedic Surgery, Children's Hospital Boston, Boston, Massachusetts

ASHWIN CHOWDHARY, MBBS, D ORTH, MS ORTH, MRCS
Clinical Fellow, Division of Paediatric Orthopaedics, National University Hospital, Singapore

ALLISON ELIZABETH CREPEAU, MD
Arnold Palmer Hospital for Children, Orlando, Florida

CHRISTOPHER K. EWING, DO
Western University of Health Sciences, Pomona, California

MEAGAN D. FERNANDEZ, DO
Department of Orthopaedic Surgery, Geisinger Medical Center, Danville, Pennsylvania

KEVIN R. FORD, PhD, FACSM
Division of Sports Medicine, Cincinnati Children's Hospital Medical Center; Department of Pediatrics, College of Medicine, University of Cincinnati, Cincinnati, Ohio

THEODORE J. GANLEY, MD
Sports Medicine Director, Division of Orthopaedic Surgery; The Sports Medicine Performance Centers, The Children's Hospital of Philadelphia; Associate Professor of Orthopaedic Surgery, The University of Pennsylvania School of Medicine, Philadelphia, Pennsylvania

BENJAMIN L. GRAY, MD
Resident Physician, Department of Orthopaedic Surgery, Washington University School of Medicine, St Louis, Missouri

NATHAN L. GRIMM, MD
Intermountain Orthopaedics, Boise, Idaho; University of Utah School of Medicine, Salt Lake City, Utah

TIMOTHY E. HEWETT, PhD, FACSM
Division of Sports Medicine, Cincinnati Children's Hospital Medical Center; Department of Pediatrics, College of Medicine, University of Cincinnati; Departments of Physiology and Cell Biology, Orthopaedic Surgery, Family Medicine and Biomedical Engineering, The Ohio State University Sports Health & Performance Institute, The Ohio State University, Cincinnati, Ohio

DESTIN E. HILL, MD
Sports Medicine Fellow, American Sports Medicine Institute, Birmingham, Alabama

VICTOR M. HO-FUNG, MD
Attending Radiologist, Department of Radiology, The Children's Hospital of Philadelphia, Philadelphia, Pennsylvania

JAMES H.P. HUI, MBBS, FRCS, MD
Associate Professor and Head, Division of Paediatric Orthopaedics, National University Hospital, Singapore

CAMILO JAIMES, MD
Research Assistant, Department of Radiology, The Children's Hospital of Philadelphia, Philadelphia, Pennsylvania

DIEGO JARAMILLO, MD, MPH
Radiologist-in-Chief and Van Alen Chair, Department of Radiology, The Children's Hospital of Philadelphia, Philadelphia, Pennsylvania

MADELYN F. KLUGMAN
Division of Sports Medicine, Cincinnati Children's Hospital Medical Center, Cincinnati, Ohio; Byram Hills High School, Armonk, New York

MININDER S. KOCHER, MD, MPH
Associate Director, Division of Sports Medicine, Children's Hospital Boston; Associate Professor of Orthopaedic Surgery, Harvard Medical School, Boston, Massachusetts

LISA M. KRUSE, MD
Resident Physician, Department of Orthopaedic Surgery, Washington University School of Medicine, St Louis, Missouri

J. TODD LAWRENCE, MD, PhD
Division of Orthopaedic Surgery, The Children's Hospital of Philadelphia, Philadelphia, Pennsylvania

MEGAN M. MAY, MD
Division of Sports Medicine, The Ohio State University, Columbus, Ohio

LYLE J. MICHELI, MD
Director, Division of Sports Medicine, Children's Hospital Boston, Boston, Massachusetts

MATTHEW D. MILEWSKI, MD
Division of Orthopaedic Surgery, Children's Hospital of Los Angeles, Los Angeles, California

GREGORY D. MYER, PhD, FACSM, CSCS
Division of Sports Medicine, Cincinnati Children's Hospital Medical Center; Department of Pediatrics and Orthopaedic Surgery, College of Medicine, University of Cincinnati; Departments of Physiology and Cell Biology, Orthopaedic Surgery, Family Medicine and Biomedical Engineering, The Ohio State University Sports Health & Performance Institute, The Ohio State University, Cincinnati, Ohio; Departments of Athletic Training, Sports Orthopaedics, and Pediatric Science, Rocky Mountain University of Health Professions, Provo, Utah

ADAM Y. NASREDDINE, MA
Research Coordinator, Department of Orthopaedic Surgery, Children's Hospital Boston, Boston, Massachusetts

GEORGE A. PALETTA Jr, MD
The Orthopedic Center of St. Louis, Chesterfield, Missouri

KEVIN G. SHEA, MD
Intermountain Orthopaedics, Boise, Idaho; University of Utah School of Medicine, Salt Lake City, Utah

ERIC J. WALL, MD
Division of Orthopaedic Surgery, Cincinnati Children's Hospital Medical Center,
Cincinnati, Ohio

RICK W. WRIGHT, MD
Professor, Residency Director, and Co-Chief Sports Medicine, Department of
Orthopaedic Surgery, Washington University School of Medicine, St Louis, Missouri

Contents

> There has been a recent trend toward more systematic, sport-specific, high-intensity physical training in children. However, there is little scientific knowledge regarding both potential benefits and hazards associated with this approach. Concurrently, an exponential increase in the number of overweight and obese children worldwide has been observed, and poor physical fitness has been identified as a primary factor contributing to the epidemic of childhood obesity. Despite this dichotomy of behavior patterns affecting the world's youth—too much or too little physical training—there is a paucity of science-based information guiding our decision making about training children and child athletes.

> With childhood obesity rates rising in most developed countries, encouraging outdoor play and sports participation may be one of several solutions for this problem. However, with the increased youth sport participation seen over the past 10 years, there has also been a need to monitor the risks of participation within this unique population. Unfortunately, only a few well-designed epidemiologic surveillance studies have been able to conduct thus far. This report focused on the injuries seen in 9 major sports played at the high school level: boys' football, soccer, basketball, baseball, and wrestling and girls' soccer, basketball, volleyball, and softball.

Anterior cruciate ligament reconstruction in the pediatric population can be performed with use of either autograft or allograft tissue. The short-term outcomes of reconstruction with nonirradiated allograft tissue are not significantly different from those with autograft tissue. Failure rates with irradiated allograft tissue, however, are significantly higher. Potential long-term donor site morbidity includes kneeling pain after harvest of autograft bone-patellar tendon-bone and knee flexor strength deficits after harvest of autograft hamstring tendons. The risk of viral and bacterial transmission from allograft tissue is very low, but not negligible. Careful donor screening and aseptic processing cannot eliminate this risk.

Treatment of anterior cruciate ligament (ACL) injuries in skeletally immature athletes is controversial. Whereas operative treatment places risk to the physis, nonoperative management may lead to functional instability. By performing physeal-sparing intraarticular and extraarticular iliotibial band reconstruction of the ACL, the risk of physeal injury is reduced and stability of the knee is restored. This article reviews the indications for iliotibial band reconstruction of the ACL in the skeletally immature athlete, surgical technique, pitfalls, and results of treatment.

Complete transphyseal reconstruction of the anterior cruciate ligament in prepubescent, skeletally immature patients must be done using a soft tissue hamstring autograft that spans or traverses the physes and with attention to the principles of tight tunnel fit, use of 0.5-mm incremental reamers with low speed and high torque, creation of a long, central tibial tunnel, avoidance of oblique femoral tunnels, and fixation proximal to the femoral physis and distal to the tibial physis. Reconstruction using these principles offers predictable outcomes of good stability and a high return to preinjury level of function with low risk for iatrogenic physeal injury.

A child's growth plate is at risk for injury during a standard "adult-style" transphyseal ACL reconstruction. Unfortunately, children who tear their

ACL and return to sports without surgery are at an extremely high risk for recurrent instability episodes. This frequently causes permanent damage to articular and meniscal cartilage that can lead to osteoarthritis. More recent "all-epiphyseal" techniques of anatomic ACL reconstruction in which the graft, the tunnels, and the fixation devices do not cross the growth plate may be the safest way to prevent a growth disturbance in a very young child.

An increase in the incidence of anterior cruciate ligament (ACL) injuries in skeletally immature athletes has led to an increase in reconstructions in this population. Once the decision for operative management has been made, the surgeon must decide with the patient and their family the optimal surgical procedure. In addition to traditional techniques for ACL reconstruction, there are several unique techniques that are growth plate respecting. The authors of this article offer their treatment algorithm for selecting ACL reconstruction surgical techniques in skeletally immature athletes. Very young children with wide open physes and minimal bone stock are treated with extraphyseal surgical techniques. Preadolescents are treated with all epiphyseal tunnels and all epiphyseal fixation. For patients who are adolescent/post pubescent but with significant femoral growth remaining, the senior author performs a hybrid technique with all epiphyseal femoral tunnel placement centered in the ACL footprint with a transphyseal tibial tunnel. For adolescent/post pubescent patients, transphyseal reconstruction is performed with the soft tissue graft only at the level of the physes and fixation adjacent to but not at the level of the physes. Advances in surgical techniques, including all epiphyseal methods, have allowed for placement of ACL grafts at the native anatomic footprint in both pre and post adolescent athletes. Incorporating these surgical techniques into comprehensive rehabilitation/prevention programs maximizes the young athlete's ability to return to healthy fitness and high level activities in a safe, timely manner.

Anterior cruciate ligament injuries in the pediatric and adolescent population are no longer the rare injury that they once were. Anterior cruciate ligament reconstruction has become increasing more common in skeletally immature patients because of increased rates of participation in organized sports as well as increased ability to diagnose these injuries. Although younger patients may pursue surgery with the short-term goal of returning to sports quickly, physicians and parents primarily wish to help them stay active, healthy, and safe in terms of minimizing or the risk of further injury.

VISIT THE CLINICS ONLINE!

Access your subscription at:
www.theclinics.com

Foreword

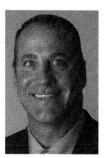

Mark D. Miller, MD
Consulting Editor

Pediatric ACL injuries. If this subject appeared 20 years ago when I coauthored two articles in a *Clinics in Sports Medicine* issue on Anterior Cruciate Ligament Injuries guest edited by a very young-looking Freddie Fu (and he still looks young), then it would have only been one article. However, it didn't even get that—and now we have dedicated an entire issue to Pediatric ACL injuries . . . Wow! Twenty years ago, a midsubstance ACL injury in a child was almost unheard of—now it is commonplace. Is this because we missed something, or is it because athletes are taking on faster and more aggressive sports earlier and earlier? Probably both, but it is true that these injuries, which remain a significant challenge, are becoming increasingly common and demand solutions. This, despite the fact that only recently have we solved (or have we?) the problem with adult ACL reconstruction with anatomic techniques, championed by, you guessed it, Dr Freddie Fu.

Dr Ted Ganley from Children's Hospital of Philadelphia (affectionately referred to as CHOP in the orthopedic world) has assembled an all-star roster of surgeons familiar with pediatric ACL injuries to bring us up to date on the challenges and (hopefully) solutions for Pediatric ACL injuries. The issue thoroughly covers controversies regarding nonoperative versus operative management, imaging, graft choices, injury prevention, rehabilitation, epidemiology, and various surgical techniques. This is an important issue, not only because these injuries are on the rise, but because these patients have so much longevity. And . . . as the saying goes, "nothing spoils good results like long-term follow-up."

Mark D. Miller, MD
S. Ward Casscells Professor of Orthopaedic Surgery
University of Virginia
Team Physician, James Madison University
400 Ray C. Hunt Drive, Suite 330
Charlottesville, VA 22908-0159, USA

E-mail address:
mdm3p@virginia.edu

Clin Sports Med 30 (2011) xiii
doi:10.1016/j.csm.2011.08.005
0278-5919/11/$ – see front matter © 2011 Elsevier Inc. All rights reserved.

Preface: ACL Injuries in the Young Athlete: A Focus on Prevention and Treatment

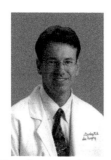

Theodore J. Ganley, MD
Guest Editor

This issue of *Clinics in Sports Medicine* addresses the topic of ACL injury in the young athlete. Sports have provided casual and elite level young athletes benefits in terms of enjoyment, camaraderie, and physical gains in strength, endurance, and flexibility. Sports also aid in the development of positive fitness habits. Unfortunately, increased training intensity and time, year-round sports, and early exposure to more competitive high demand sports have led to an increase in injuries including ACL ruptures. Significant progress has been made, however, in understanding the incidence of this injury as well as novel treatment modalities, rehabilitation, and injury prevention.

In this issue of *Clinics in Sports Medicine*, leading experts have written state-of-the-art articles in areas related to ACL epidemiology, imaging, ACL avulsion fractures, partial injuries, graft choices, surgical techniques, algorithms of treatment, and rehabilitation. Also included are articles that address training, health promotion and performance, injury prevention, and stopping sports injuries in young athletes. These articles address emerging treatment options and highlight areas of ongoing investigation.

To help young athletes and their families better understand some of the fundamental questions as well as more complex issues surrounding ACL injuries, Dr Carey and I have provided a series of questions and answers as an addition to this preface (**Box 1**).

I am indebted to the senior, corresponding authors of each article, who were selected because they have dedicated their life's work to developing better ways to evaluate, treat, and prevent sports injuries and specifically ACL injuries in this unique population of patients. I am also grateful to the aspiring junior colleagues who have participated as coauthors.

Clin Sports Med 30 (2011) xv–xviii
doi:10.1016/j.csm.2011.08.006
0278-5919/11/$ – see front matter © 2011 Elsevier Inc. All rights reserved.

sportsmed.theclinics.com

Box 1
Questions and answers about ACL injury and ACL surgery
Information for young athletes and their families

Theodore J. Ganley, MD, and James L. Carey, MD, MPH

What is the ACL?	The anterior cruciate ligament or ACL is a tether in the center of the knee that prevents excessive forward translation and rotation of the shin bone. The ACL provides athletes with a stable knee while playing sports.
Why does the ACL tear?	The ACL can withstand a certain amount of force and when that force is exceeded it tears or ruptures. ACL injuries most commonly occur during explosive pivoting maneuvers or traumatic collisions. The ACL is like the stop on the tracks beneath a kitchen drawer. When the drawer is pulled with too much force, the stop can be broken causing the drawer to fall to the floor.
What steps are necessary to confirm that the ACL is injured?	A young athlete will sometimes report a popping sensation at the time of injury. Immediately after the injury, the knee swells over 24 to 48 hours. This gradual swelling is analogous to a dripping faucet. On physical examination, a knee with an ACL injury will demonstrate abnormal motion when the examiner pulls on the shin bone. Magnetic resonance imaging can be used along with the history and physical examination to confirm that the ACL has been torn.
Does the ACL heal itself?	The ACL does not heal itself for a few reasons. First, the ruptured ends of the ACL can be shortened and frayed with multiple strands. It can have the appearance of a firecracker after it has exploded. Second, the fluid in the knee joint can keep the ends from healing. An analogy is that a small cut on your hand heals well after forming a clot and then a scab. However, this same cut does not heal if it is kept under running water that continually washes the clot away.
Can I just participate in all of my sports without an ACL?	There are two reasons that returning to sports without limitations is not considered "medically advisable." Without explosive capabilities, athletes involved in running, jumping, and pivoting sports cannot make meaningful contributions to their teams. The ACL is also the primary stabilizer of the knee and giving way episodes from these sports can lead to cartilage injuries including the joint surfaces and the menisci, which are secondary stabilizers of the knee.

Is surgery required?	This decision between young athletes, their parents, and health care providers is a shared one based on the individual issues of the athlete and their entire family. In general, however, surgical treatment is considered the gold standard method of treatment of ACL ruptures in young athletes.
What is surgical reconstruction?	It is the process by which the ruptured ligament is replaced with a new ligament.
Why do surgeries differ between preadolescent and adolescent athletes?	There are a number of fundamental differences including the size of the knee, the size and shape of growth plates, as well as the ability of much younger athletes to gain muscle bulk. Variations in surgical techniques help accommodate for closing growth plates in older adolescents and for wide open growth plates in younger patients.
Where does the ligament come from?	Autograft tissue comes from the injured athlete. Allograft tissue comes from a cadaver, meaning someone who passed away and donated their tissues to others.
When can I return to play?	Young athletes return to play after regaining full motion and strength. In addition, a balance training program is completed as part of rehabilitation. Many orthopedic surgeons performing ACL surgery also require their young athletes to wait a minimum of 6 months (or even 9 months in younger patients) between the date of ACL reconstruction and the date of return to play.
Will I require a brace?	The results of orthopedic studies do not provide a clear consensus to mandate or eliminate the use of postsurgical bracing in adolescent athletes. This decision is decided on an individual basis accounting for the combination of injuries sustained and for the extreme nature of certain sports. While the literature is limited, orthopedic physicians most often prescribe functional knee bracing in the event of a partial ACL rupture or in an ACL-deficient knee in a young athlete planning for a delayed reconstruction.
Is there a chance of re-injury?	The chance of rupturing the new ACL graft is on the order of 5%. Of note, the chance of rupturing the ACL in the uninjured knee is estimated to be on the order of 10% The goals of more recent motion, strength and rehabilitation/prevention programs is to minimize the risk of injury. Noting that the injury risk to the affected knee is half of that of the unaffected knee, strengthening/prevention programs should also address and focus on the unaffected knee to eliminate or minimize future injury. The authors of this issue of *Clinics in Sports Medicine* provide their patients with the comprehensive postoperative and preventive programs described.

Courtesy of T. Ganley, MD, Philadelphia, PA

I am hopeful that the readers appreciate and enjoy the scientific content provided by the contributors. I believe that this collection of exceptional articles will serve as a valuable resource for medical professionals, athletes, and their families. It is a privilege to have been asked to recruit and edit articles from this internationally renowned group of colleagues whose efforts have made this issue successful.

Theodore J. Ganley, MD
Division of Orthopaedic Surgery
The Children's Hospital of Philadelphia
34th and Civic Center Boulevard
Philadelphia, PA 19104, USA

Erratum

An error was made in the July issue of *Clinics in Sports Medicine*, Volume 30, Number 3, in the article titled "The International Athlete—Advances in Management of Jet Lag Disorder and Anti-Doping Policy" by Daniel Herman, MD, PhD, John M. MacKnight, MD, Amy E. Stromwall, MD, and Dilaawar J. Mistry, MD, ATC, on pages 641–659. Page 641 did not list the correct corresponding author address, which is Departments of Athletics and Physical Medicine and Rehabilitation, University of Virginia Health System, 545 Ray C. Hunt Drive, Suite 240, PO Box 801004, Charlottesville, VA 22908-1004, USA.

The author affiliation footnotes were also listed incorrectly for Drs Stromwall and Mistry and should have been listed as:

AMY E. STROMWALL, MD
Summit Orthopedics Ltd, 310 Smith Avenue North, Saint Paul, MN 55102, USA; U.S.A. Swimming, 1 Olympic Plaza, Colorado Springs, CO 80909, USA

DILAAWAR J. MISTRY, MD, ATC
Departments of Athletics and Physical Medicine and Rehabilitation, University of Virginia Health System, 545 Ray C. Hunt Drive, Suite 240, PO Box 801004, Charlottesville, VA 22908-1004, USA

Clin Sports Med 30 (2011) xix
doi:10.1016/j.csm.2011.08.004
0278-5919/11/$ – see front matter © 2011 Elsevier Inc. All rights reserved.

Training the Child Athlete for Prevention, Health Promotion, and Performance: How Much Is Enough, How Much Is Too Much?

Cordelia W. Carter, MD, Lyle J. Micheli, MD*

KEYWORDS
• Child athlete • Training • Injury • Overuse

INTRODUCTION

In recent years, there has been a global trend toward more systematic, sport-specific, high-intensity training in younger children. Despite this increasingly common practice, there is little scientific knowledge regarding the potential benefits of highly focused, intensive training for the participating child, and perhaps more worrisome, little systematic study of the possible hazards this type of training might present to the child's developing mind and body.[1] At the same time, there has been an exponential increase in the number of children worldwide who are overweight and frankly obese.[2] Increasing physical activity levels in this cohort of children and adolescents has been a cornerstone of many public health interventions designed to fight the epidemic of obesity, yet not all have been successful.[3] Sadly, despite this dichotomy of potentially hazardous behavior patterns affecting the world's youth—too much or little training—there is a paucity of science-based information guiding our decision making about training children and the child athlete.

Guidelines for physical activity in children were first established by the American College of Sports Medicine in 1988[2] with the goals of optimizing bone health, muscular strength, flexibility, and general health. The initial recommendation of the convened expert panel was for 20 to 30 minutes of vigorous exercise daily. Subsequent recommendations established in 1994 by the International Consensus Conference on Physical Activity Guidelines for Adolescents were also based largely on expert opinion.[4] With their dual goals of promoting physical and psychological health and well-being during adolescence as well as enhancing future health, this

Division of Sports Medicine, Children's Hospital Boston, 319 Longwood Avenue, Boston, MA 02115, USA
* Corresponding author.
E-mail address: michelilyle@aol.com

Clin Sports Med 30 (2011) 679–690
doi:10.1016/j.csm.2011.06.004
0278-5919/11/$ – see front matter © 2011 Elsevier Inc. All rights reserved.

panel concluded that (1) "all adolescents should be physically active daily or nearly every day" and that (2) "adolescents should engage in three or more sessions per week of activities that last 20 minutes or more at a time and require moderate to vigorous levels of exertion." Subsequent proposals (eg, that of the Health Education Authority in the United Kingdom) increased the recommended amount of daily activity for children to 60 minutes of at least moderate intensity activity, and this recommendation has had some support in the scientific literature.[5,6] However, although researchers continue to hone in on the optimal frequency, duration, and intensity of physical activity for children and adolescents, there is little information regarding what constitutes excessive or potentially harmful training as well as what the effects—both beneficial and deleterious—of high-intensity, sport-specialization may be.

COMPONENTS OF TRAINING
Cardiovascular Training

Cardiovascular training, or endurance training, may be defined as a "structured exercise program that is sustained for a sufficient length of time with sufficient intensity and frequency to induce an improvement in aerobic fitness."[7] Aerobic fitness is influenced by several factors such as genetics, age, gender, and fat mass, but is largely determined by the frequency, duration, and intensity of physical activity performed over time. Although early studies of child and adolescent athletes failed to demonstrate a significant "trainability" to children's cardiovascular systems, more recent research has shown that training children maximally does in fact demonstrate a training effect, as evidenced by changes in pulse rate and measured peak oxygen uptake (VO_{2max}).[8] Elite, "trained" young athletes, as described by Armstrong and Barker,[7] have higher VO_{2max} than their untrained peers with faster VO_2 kinetic responses to changes in exercise intensity. In fact, according to 1 author, children's maximal oxygen consumption typically improves by 5% to 6% in response to aerobic training, with the magnitude of change, depending on initial fitness level ("pretrained" athletes demonstrate smaller effects than their untrained peers).[9] There is evidence, too, that this training effect can be lost and that aerobic fitness decreases to a level close to 30 mLO_2/min/kg in children if they are sedentary, regardless of their genetic profile.[10] The existence of a "maturational threshold" below which children are not trainable has not been established,[7] and current wisdom holds that young people can indeed benefit from endurance training, albeit at a higher relative intensity than is required in the adult.

Based on their review of the available scientific literature, the International Olympic Committee's Medical Commission on training the elite child athlete recommended both aerobic (3–4 sessions per week of 40–60 minutes at an intensity of 85%–90% of maximum heart rate) and anaerobic (intensity >90% maximum heart rate and <30 seconds' duration) training as part of a complete and optimal training program.[1]

Resistance Training

Resistance training has been defined as a "method of physical conditioning that involves the progressive use of a wide range of resistive loads, different movement velocities and a variety of training modalities including weight machines, free weights . . . elastic bands, medicine balls and plyometrics."[11] Resistance training was traditionally discouraged for children and adolescents as a result of unfounded concerns that it was unsafe for the skeletally immature population.[12] However, there is now an abundance of scientific literature demonstrating that resistance training is not only safe for the child and adolescent athlete, but is routinely associated with increased muscle strength, and in fact may play a role in the prevention of sports-related injuries.[11] Faigenbaum and Myer[11] recently reviewed the available literature on resistance training in children and adolescents, reporting on 27 studies that employed a resistance training intervention in youth aged 6 to 18 years. Only 3 injuries were reported in this group: (1) Shoulder pain that resolved with 1 week of rest; (2) a shoulder strain that resulted in 1 missed training session; and (3) thigh pain that resolved with 5 minutes of rest. The estimated injury rates for these studies were 0.176, 0.053, and 0.055 per 100 participant-hours, respectively, (compared with rugby, for example, which has been reported to have an injury rate of 0.800 per 100 participant-hours[11]). Although these authors report upon several case studies of physeal injury related to resistance training, they note that these injuries were almost exclusively the result of improper technique, inappropriate training load, or lack of qualified supervision.

There is good available evidence demonstrating the efficacy of resistance training in child and adolescent athletes for improving muscle strength, with strength gains of up to 74% reported in 1 study after 8 weeks of progressive resistance training.[13] As summarized by Faigenbaum and colleagues,[13] 2 meta-analyses evaluating the effectiveness of resistance training in youth demonstrated a significant positive association between resistance training and strength gains, with effect sizes of 0.57 and 0.75, respectively. It is now almost universally accepted that resistance training, when performed under the close supervision of a qualified instructor, using appropriate training equipment, and a stepwise progression of loads and skills, is safe and effective for the young athlete. As a result, the International Olympic Committee's Medical Commission recommends the inclusion of resistance training in the repertoire of the elite child athlete, and concludes that "an effective and safe strength training program . . . includes a minimum of 2 to 3 sessions per week with 3 sets, at an intensity of between 50 and 85% of the 1 repetition maximal."[1]

Flexibility Training

It is an oft-observed phenomenon that children's flexibility decreases as they age, potentially increasing the stress across major joints (eg, knees, hips) and resulting in a host of musculoskeletal complaints including patellofemoral pain, iliotibial band syndrome, and low back pain. Additionally, it is widely accepted that sports-related injuries tend to occur more commonly during the time of peak growth velocity and some component of this increased risk may be attributed to the relative tightening of major joint-spanning muscle groups whose longitudinal growth has failed to keep pace with that of the adjacent bones.[14] As a result, flexibility training—including adequate warm-up, stretching, and cool-down sessions—should be a critical component of the young athlete's training regimen.

TRAINING BENEFITS

There are 4 primary acknowledged advantages to training the child athlete: (1) Health promotion; (2) injury prevention; (3) psychological benefits; and (4) performance enhancement.

Health Promotion

Cardiovascular health
As childhood obesity has become more prevalent worldwide, public health initiatives have focused increasingly on weight management—targeting "fatness" in children and adolescents—as a means of improving health. However, several groups of researchers have recently determined that it is not simply obesity that puts children at

risk for developing long-term health problems such as cardiovascular disease and the metabolic syndrome (a precursor to type II diabetes mellitus characterized by abdominal adiposity, dyslipidemia, hypertension, and altered glucose metabolism). Rather, poor aerobic fitness is a significant marker for the development of cardiovascular risk factors in childhood independent of weight or body mass index (BMI).

In a recent study performed by Resalund and associates,[15] a cohort of 9-year-old Norwegian schoolchildren was evaluated for the presence of cardiovascular risk factors—homeostasis model assessment score (a measure of altered glucose metabolism), waist circumference, triglyceride level, systolic blood pressure, total cholesterol/high-density lipoprotein ratio, and aerobic fitness as defined by peak oxygen consumption (VO_{2peak}).[15] These authors reported a significant association between the clustered cardiovascular risk factors and low fitness (as measured by VO_{2peak} on a treadmill protocol.) They concluded that aerobic fitness is an important marker of health in children and that fitness testing may play an important role in childhood health assessments.

These findings dovetail with earlier work published by Andersen and co-workers,[5] who demonstrated that clustered risk factors for cardiovascular disease—systolic blood pressure, triglyceride level, total cholesterol/high-density lipoprotein ratio, and insulin resistance—had a significant inverse association with physical activity level, as measured by accelerometer in 9- and 15-year-old European children. These authors calculate that as much as 90 minutes of physical activity daily might be necessary to prevent the clustering of cardiovascular risk factors in children. In a follow-up study, Andersen and associates[3] noted that aerobic fitness (VO_{2max}), as measured by a cycle ergometer test, had an independent negative association with clustered cardiovascular risk factors in children.

In the European Youth Heart Study, Adegboye and colleagues[10] evaluated the same population of 9- and 15-year-old European schoolchildren using the same known cardiovascular risk factors and measuring aerobic fitness by VO_{2peak} relative to bodyweight on the aforementioned cycle test. These authors used receiver operating characteristic analysis to determine fitness "cutoff points" that would identify those children at risk for cardiovascular disease.

Each of these studies highlights the importance of incorporating fitness testing routinely into pediatric health screening as a means of identifying children and adolescents that are likely to develop risk factors for cardiovascular disease and the metabolic syndrome. Because these cardiovascular risk factors have been shown to reliably "track" into adolescence and adulthood, it seems logical that identifying children at risk for cardiovascular disease as a result of poor fitness and implementing targeted early intervention programs might prove to be a successful strategy for the long-term prevention of cardiovascular disease. In fact, a recent Cochrane review of school-based physical activity programs found a consistent association between physical activity in the school setting and improved VO_{2max} and serum cholesterol levels.[16]

Finally, some recent studies have focused on the role of resistance training, rather than simply aerobic fitness levels, in mediating cardiovascular risk factors in children and adolescents. There is some evidence to support an association between resistance training and improved glucose metabolism and decreased body fat in adolescents.[13] However, the association between resistance training and blood pressure, lipid profile, and other measures of metabolic health in youth remains unclear at this time.

Bone health

Both the mass (quantity) and structure (quality) of bone play a significant role in determining its strength, which in turn is important for determining the relative risk of fracture. Importantly, the growing skeleton in children and adolescents is supremely responsive to mechanical strain placed on it by weight-bearing physical activity, adapting to this stress by increasing overall bone mass. In fact, the adolescent skeleton is capable of vast quantities of bone mineral accrual, with an estimated 26% of the total adult bone mass gained in merely 2 years during the adolescent peak of bone mineral accumulation (this occurs at 12.5 years of age in girls and 14.1 years of age in boys).[17] Peak bone mass is generally achieved in the young adult years, and gradually declines over time. Thus, because the young skeletal system is primed to respond to the osteogenic influence of weight-bearing physical activity by increasing bone formation, some authors have viewed this age as a "window of opportunity" during which physical activity might be used to build bony stores and theoretically protect against future fracture.[17] It should be noted that gains in bone mass have been observed for aerobic weight-bearing activity, such as running, as well as for resistance training activities, including strength training and plyometrics.[11]

In their review of the association between physical activity and bone health, Boreham and McKay[17] detail various observational, epidemiologic, and experimental studies of children and adolescents that support the association between physical activity and increased bone mass in this population. Although these authors caution that cessation of physical activity may well result in a loss of the observed gains in bone strength over time, there is no doubt that physical activity during childhood and adolescence has a positive effect on bone health. They conclude that public health efforts aimed at maximizing the "bone bank" during the adolescent peak of bone mineral accrual remain a primary strategy for fracture reduction and suggest that future research should focus on determining the optimal "dose" of physical activity for maximally enhancing bone strength.[17]

Injury Prevention

There is good evidence to support the assertion of a positive relationship between training and injury prevention in the child and adolescent athlete.[11,13,14] The area that has perhaps received the most recent attention in the scientific literature has been the prevention of anterior cruciate ligament (ACL) injuries in adolescent females athletes through the implementation of various neuromuscular, plyometric, and proprioceptive training programs.[18] Myriad studies have identified potentially modifiable factors placing young women at risk for this injury, including extended hip and knee-joint postures on landing from a jump; decreased hamstring-to-quadriceps strength ratios; overall poor physical conditioning; low core, trunk, and hip strength; and increased valgus knee moments with landing and squatting.[19]

The majority of interventional studies have utilized a combination of plyometrics, proprioceptive training, strengthening, stretching, aerobic training, and risk awareness training to effect changes in these potentially modifiable risk factors and ultimately decrease the rate of noncontact ACL injuries in female athletes. Most of these studies have reported a positive association between training interventions and decreased ACL injuries in these athletes.[20–22] Hewitt and associates, for example, used a 6-week neuromuscular training program comprised of stretching, plyometrics, and weight training to investigate its effect on the rate of serious knee injury including noncontact ACL injury.[20] These authors reported a rate of serious knee injury as much as 3.6 times higher in the untrained group; they additionally noted that whereas 5 untrained female athletes sustained injuries to the ACL, not a single female athlete in the trained group sustained a similar injury.[20]

In a subsequent study, Mandelbaum and colleagues investigated the efficacy of their Prevent Injury and Enhance Performance Program for preventing noncontact ACL injuries in adolescent female soccer players.[21] The experimental group received videotaped instruction on the performance of 3 basic warm-up activities, 5 stretching techniques, 3 strengthening exercises, 5 plyometric exercises, and 3 soccer-specific agility drills; emphasis was placed throughout on using proper biomechanical technique. Athletes in both the experimental and matched control groups were then followed for 2 years, and data concerning athletic exposure and ACL injuries was collected. Significantly, these authors reported 6 ACL injuries in the trained group, compared with 67 in the untrained group, corresponding to an average decrease in ACL injury of more than 70%.[21]

Other authors have examined the association between the implementation of neuromuscular training programs and the rates of overall injury (not specifically ACL injury) in youth sports.[22–25] Heidt and co-workers,[22] for example, looked at 300 adolescent female soccer players, randomly selecting 42 of them to participate in a preseason training program consisting of cardiovascular training, plyometrics, strength, and flexibility training and sport-cord drills over a 7-week period. Over the course of 1 year, they found that the untrained group had sustained significantly more injuries (33.7% vs 14.3%), the vast majority of which occurred in the knee and ankle. Additionally, 8 athletes in the untrained group sustained ACL injury versus only 1 in the trained group, although this finding failed to achieve significance. Olsen and colleagues[23] investigated the effects of a similar neuromuscular training program on Norwegian handball players and found a significant protective effect of training for all acute knee or ankle injuries (48 injuries occurred in the intervention group versus 81 in the control group). They additionally found a significantly greater number of ligamentous knee injuries in the untrained group. Finally, Emery and Meeuwisse[24] published the results of their randomized, controlled trial investigating the effect of training on injury rates in youth. These authors, too, reported a significant difference in injury rates between the trained and untrained cohorts; they additionally noted trends toward decreased ankle and knee sprains specifically in the trained group, although these did not achieve significance.

Importantly, injury prevention during sports participation is not limited to the highly trained athlete; in fact, there is good data demonstrating that youth with increased BMIs have a significantly higher risk of sustaining a sports-related injury than their normal-weight peers. In a review of the available literature on obesity and injury, McHugh[26] reported that in 11 of the 13 studies included in his analysis, a higher BMI and/or high percentage of body fat were associated with an increased risk of sports-related injury (specifically ankle sprains, medial collateral ligament tears and dental injuries). The reported increases in injury risk ranged from 1.4 to 3.9 times the risk identified for the normal-weight control groups. Proposed mechanisms for this finding in overweight and obese children include poor postural control (leading to problems with balance and coordination), poor physical fitness (associated with muscle fatigue and subsequent injury), and low pre-participation physical activity levels (associated with impaired neuromuscular and motor learning). Proposed interventions include improving overall physical fitness and neuromuscular control through targeted cardiovascular and resistance training regimens. There is additional evidence to suggest that balance training programs in the obese adolescent population are successful at decreasing the risk of sports-related ankle sprains.[19]

Psychological Benefits

There is a widely held belief that physical activity is associated with positive changes in mental and emotional well-being, and there is some scientific evidence in support of this supposition. However, studies of this association are frequently cross-sectional and some are quasi-experimental in nature and so drawing firm conclusions about the causality of this relationship is a practice fraught with problems. That said, 2 recent meta-analyses have suggested significant associations between physical activity and several different indices of mental health. In 2005, Strong and colleageus[6] convened an expert panel to "review and evaluate available evidence on the influence of physical activity on several health and behavioral outcomes in youth aged 6–18 years." Outcomes measured included symptoms of anxiety and depression, self-concept, and academic performance. Based on the available data, these authors conclude that there is evidence to support a positive association between physical activity and lower scores on scales of anxiety and depression symptoms. Additionally, they found that children and adolescents with a strong "athletic identity" demonstrate higher levels of self-esteem, particularly in the domains of physical appearance and physical competency. Importantly, higher self-esteem may positively enhance the physical, psychological, and social adaptation of the child to the tumultuous period of adolescence.[27] Finally, Strong and associates[6] also reviewed cross-sectional and mechanistic studies evaluating the relationship between participation in physical activity and academic performance, as assessed by grade point average and standardized testing scores. These authors noted that there is a positive association between academic performance and physical activity and physical fitness; they add that physical activity has a positive influence on concentration and memory as well as on classroom behavior.[6]

In their "review of reviews," Biddle and Asare[28] examined the existing literature on the relationship between physical activity and multiple factors of mental health including depression, anxiety, self-esteem, and cognitive functioning. While again noting that these associations have only been weakly established and that rigorous prospective studies will be required to confirm their significance, these authors conclude that based on the available data, "physical activity over no intervention appears to be potentially beneficial for reduced depression."[28] Their conclusions about anxiety reduction are similar. Looking at self-esteem, they noted that each of the review articles they examined demonstrated small to moderate effect sizes of physical activity on enhanced self-esteem. Finally, they reiterated the earlier findings of Strong and co-workers[6] regarding cognitive functioning, noting that the cognitive skills of concentration and attention as well as academic achievement are all correlate with increased levels of physical activity.

Performance Enhancement

Based on the previous sections identifying clear training benefits on the cardiovascular, bone, and mental health of the child athlete, all of which may logically be associated with enhanced athletic performance, it seems reasonable to assume that this domain, too, may be positively affected by training. Additionally, there is some evidence from the ACL prevention literature demonstrating that multimodal neuromuscular training programs (which incorporate aerobic training, resistance training, and flexibility training) are effective at improving performance measures of speed, strength and power.[26] There is no question that an aerobically fit, physically strong, and mentally well-grounded child athlete will perform at the top of his game.

TRAINING CONCERNS

Although physical activity for children and adolescents has been associated with a host of previously described health and wellness benefits, sometimes there can be too much of a good thing. Just as adult athletes may suffer from overtraining syndrome, burnout, and overuse injuries, children who perform excessive amounts of high-intensity, repetitive physical activity without adequate rest or break times allotted may be susceptible to the perils of overtraining.

Although they have been better characterized in adults, overtraining syndrome and burnout have been additionally described in children. Overtraining syndrome typically presents as a constellation of symptoms including fatigue, sleep disturbances, chronic muscle and/or joint pain, elevated resting heart rate, performance decline, mood disturbances including irritability or decreased attention span, and in the child athlete, impaired academic performance as evidenced by lower grades.[29,30] Overtraining syndrome in adults is additionally associated with changes in the hypothalamic–pituitary–adrenal axis, which results in altered hormonal responses to intensive training and competition, including changes in the serum concentrations for cortisol, adrenocorticotropic hormone, prolactin, and human growth hormone. These psychological, physiologic, and hormonal changes ultimately interact to impair athletic performance.[31]

Overtraining syndrome and burnout are routinely associated with changes in an athlete's cognitive and mood profile; specifically, "burnt-out" athletes demonstrate decreased vigor and the less adaptive mood states of fatigue, confusion, depression, anger, and tension are all increased—the precise opposite mood profile of a healthy, high-functioning athlete.[29] The athlete's physiologic response to the perceived stress of continued athletic participation may then result in the aforementioned tachycardia and personality changes associated with the overtraining syndrome. This same stress response may additionally lead to increased muscle tension, narrowing of the visual field, and distractibility, which predispose these stressed, "burnt-out" athletes to sports-related injury at significantly higher rates than their appropriately trained peers.[27,29,32,33]

In addition to the acute sports-related injuries that overtrained athletes may sustain, overuse injuries are frequently associated with overtraining and burnout.[14] As described by Brenner,[30] overuse injuries are a clear physical representation of overtraining and may be defined as "microtraumatic damage to a bone, muscle, or tendon that has been subjected to repetitive stress without sufficient time to heal or undergo the natural reparative process." They can be classified into 4 stages: (1) Pain in the affected area after physical activity; (2) pain during activity, without restricting performance; (3) pain during activity that restricts performance; (4) chronic, unremitting pain, even at rest.[30]

In an excellent review of overtraining and overuse injuries in children put out by the Council on Sports Medicine and Fitness, several specific practices that potentially put young athletes at an increased risk for overuse injuries and burnout are identified.[30] These practices include participation in weekend tournaments and year-round training on multiple teams. With societal emphasis placed on early sport specialization and perfecting sport-specific skills, many child athletes find themselves participating in a single sport—for example, soccer, baseball, basketball—on multiple teams throughout the year, often traveling miles to weekend tournaments where competition can literally last all day. In the absence of appropriate breaks for physical and mental rest, these athletes are likely at increased risk for overtraining syndrome and injury.

Participation in endurance events, such as marathon running, has been identified as a possible harmful practice for children.[34] However, Brenner[30] acknowledges that although much concern has been voiced over the participation of children and adolescents in endurance events, there is actually little scientific evidence to support the claim that endurance events are harmful to the developing child. In fact, gradually progressing the child's training regimen (advancing both endurance and intensity in a stepwise fashion) is generally held to be a safe practice. Many clinicians still adhere to the "10% rule" as a training guideline, which states that "each week there should be no more than a 10% increase in the amount of training time, amount of distance covered, or number of repetitions performed in the activity."[14] As long as training progression is gradual and the child athlete is carefully monitored for signs of injury or burnout, participation in endurance events does not seem to be deleterious.

Finally, Although it is well-recognized that single-sport athletes who participate in year-round competition on multiple teams are particularly prone to overuse injuries and burnout, multisport athletes may be at risk for similar problems if they fail to get enough rest between daily activities (multiple sports, same season) or an adequate break between seasons. Poor periodization, therefore, seems to place young athletes at risk for overtraining syndrome and injury. It should be noted, however, that with sufficient rest between seasons, being a multisport athlete seems to be protective against overtraining and burnout, with some evidence demonstrating that young athletes who participate in a variety of sports sustain fewer injuries and participate in sports longer than their counterparts who specialize in a single sport at an early age.[30]

Studies to date have suggested that the prevention of sports injuries in children requires a determination of the risk factors for injury in each sport and the instrumentation of prevention strategies that take into account the special risk factors of the child athlete. Both inadequate and excessive training regimens have been identified as risk factors for injury.[35–38]

Of special interest to the physician caring for the child or adolescent athlete are the overuse or overtraining injuries specific to that cohort. The major concern with training the skeletally immature athlete is damaging the growth cartilage.[14] Injuries to the growth cartilage may be divided into articular, apophyseal, and physeal injuries. Osteochondritis dissecans lesions, which are frequently found in the knee, elbow, and ankle of physically active children and affect primarily the articular cartilage and subchondral bone, are a common sequela of overtraining. The apophyseal cartilage of the knee (Osgood–Schlatter's disease) and elbow ("little leaguer's elbow") are locations commonly affected by repetitive use, resulting in a painful traction apophysitis.[39] Additionally, the physis itself may be injured as a result of overuse: Little leaguer's shoulder and gymnast's wrist are both examples of this phenomenon. Finally, frank failure of bone as a result of repetitive loading may also be seen in the overtrained athlete. Lumbar spondylolysis, often seen in the gymnast, ballerina, or wrestler, are examples.[40]

There are 2 additional peculiarities of the child athlete that put him or her at risk for overtraining injury: Specifically, children have a well-documented increased susceptibility to the elements (especially heat exhaustion) when compared with adult athletes.[30] Ensuring the safety of the child athlete therefore requires an awareness of weather conditions and modifying training sessions to accommodate them appropriately (ie, increasing the frequency of water breaks, shortening practice time, and training during cooler hours). Children are most susceptible to sustaining a sports-related injury during the time of their peak growth velocity.[14] This is likely related to a combination of muscle imbalances resulting from asymmetric growth, relatively tightened muscles as the soft tissues lag behind the osseous structures in longitudinal growth, and decrements in proprioception and balance resulting from adjustment to rapid bony growth.

It is important to recognize that because of the extreme variability in physical and psychological maturation among children of the same chronologic age, the frequency, duration, or intensity of physical activity that is appropriate for 1 child may be frankly overwhelming, both physically and emotionally, for a same-age peer. This makes rigid prescriptive guidelines for physical activity in the child and adolescent athlete untenable; rather, each athlete must be evaluated individually and the onus lies on the athlete's coaches and parents to be aware of the signs of overtraining and burnout and to intervene in a timely fashion.

SUMMARY

With growing numbers of youth worldwide participating in athletics at ever-increasing levels of intensity, there is a clear need to establish training guidelines that would optimize athletic performance without compromising the child athlete's physical, mental, and emotional health. At the same time, there has arisen a global epidemic of childhood obesity and its associated health problems of cardiovascular disease and diabetes mellitus. Taken in this context, the mounting scientific data demonstrating positive effects of training on cardiovascular, bone, and mental health provide strong support for setting a minimal training threshold for every child.

Currently, the medical literature is inadequate to offer a universal prescription for optimally training children and child athletes and rigorous scientific investigation is needed to determine the optimal "dose–response" curve for training, as well as to establish potential minimal and maximal training thresholds. Prospective clinical studies that carefully monitor and document children's training activities in addition to the physiologic responses that are elicited—both positive and negative—are required.

In the absence of this type of data, guidelines for training the child athlete should therefore be (1) individual specific, taking into account factors such as a child's gender, age, BMI, injury history, developmental level, and skill set; (2) sport specific (Is the sport contact or noncontact? Does it require frequent repetitive motions?); and (3) context specific, with awareness of the level of play, relevant weather conditions, and season length, informing all training recommendations. Additionally, the concepts of gradual training progression—adhering to the "10%" rule—and periodization should be used to prevent injury and burnout. Perhaps most important is to remember that it is the ultimate responsibility of involved adults—coaches, parents, trainers, and teachers—to ensure the health and safety of each child.

REFERENCES

1. Mountjoy M, Armstrong N, Bizzini L, et al. IOC consensus statement on training the elite child athlete. Clin J Sport Med 2008;18:122–3.
2. American College of Sports Medicine. Physical fitness in children and youth. Med Sci Sports Exerc 1988;20:422–3.
3. Andersen LB, Sardinha LB, Froberg K, et al. Fitness, fatness and clustering of cardiovascular risk factors in children from Denmark, Estonia and Portugal: The European Youth Heart Study. Int J Pediatr Obes 2008;3(Suppl. 1):58–66.
4. Sallis JF, Patrick K. Physical activity guidelines for adolescents: consensus statement. Pediatr Exerc Sci 1994;6:302–14.
5. Andersen LB, Harro H, Sardinha LB, et al. Physical activity and clustered cardiovascular risk in children: a cross-sectional study (The European Youth Heart Study). Lancet 2006;368:299–304.

6. Strong WB, Malina RM, Blimke CJ, et al. Evidence based physical activity for school-age youth. J Pediatr 2005;146:732–7.
7. Armstrong N, Barker AR. Endurance training and elite young athletes. Med Sport Sci 2011;56:59–83.
8. Mathews KA, Stoney CM. Influence of sex and age on cardiovascular responses during stress. Psychosom Med 1988;50:46–56.
9. Tomkinson G. Aerobic fitness thresholds for cardio metabolic health in children and adolescents. Br J Sports Med 2011;45:686–7.
10. Adegboye AR, Anderssen SA, Froberg K, et al. Recommended aerobic fitness level for metabolic health in children and adolescents: a study of diagnostic accuracy. Br J Sports Med 2011;45:722–8.
11. Faigenbaum AD, Myer GD. Resistance training among young athletes: safety, efficacy and injury prevention effects. Br J Sports Med 2010;44:56–63.
12. American Academy of Pediatrics. Weight training and weight lifting: information for the pediatrician. Phys Sports Med 1983;11;157–61.
13. Faigenbaum AD, Kraemer WJ, Blimkie CJ, et al. Youth resistance training: updated position statement paper from the national strength and conditioning association. J Strength Cond Res 2009;23:S60–79.
14. Smith AD, Andrish JT, Micheli LJ. The prevention of sports injuries of children and adolescents. Med Sci Sports Exerc 1993;25:1–7.
15. Resalund GK, Mamen A, Boreham C, et al. Cardiovascular risk factor clustering and its association with fitness in nine-year-old rural Norwegian children. Scand J Med Sci Sports 2010;20:e112–20.
16. Dobbins M, DeCorby K, Robeson P, et al. School-based physical activity programs for promoting physical activity and fitness in children and adolescents aged 6–18. Cochrane Database of Systematic Reviews. 2009;1:CD007651.
17. Boreham C, McKay H. Physical activity and bone health. Br J Sports Med, in press.
18. Renstrom P, Ljungqvist A, Arendt E, et al. Noncontact ACL injuries in female athletes: an International Olympic Committee Current Concepts Statement. Br J Sports Med 2008;42;394–412.
19. Alentorn-Geli E, Myer GD, Silvers HJ, et al. Prevention of non-contact anterior cruciate ligament injuries in soccer players. Part 2: a review of prevention programs aimed to modify risk factors and to reduce injury rates. Knee Surg Sports Traumatol Arthrosc 2009;17:859–79.
20. Hewitt TE, Lindenfield TN, Riccobene JV, et al. The effect of neuromuscular training on the incidence of knee injury in female athletes. Am J Sports Med 1999;27:699–706.
21. Mandelbaum BR, Silvers HJ, Watanabe DS, et al. Effectiveness of a neuromuscular and proprioceptive training program in preventing anterior cruciate ligament injuries in female athletes. 2 year follow-up. Am J Sports Med 2005;33:1003–10.
22. Heidt RS, Sweeterman LM, Carlonas RL, et al. Avoidance of soccer injuries with preseason conditioning. Am J Sports Med 2000;28:659–62.
23. Olsen O, Myklebust G, Engebretsen L, et al. Exercises to prevent lower limb injuries in youth sports: cluster randomised controlled trial. BMJ 2005;330:220.
24. Emery CA, Meeuwisse WH. The effectiveness of a neuromuscular prevention strategy to reduce injuries in youth soccer: a cluster-randomised controlled trial. Br J Sports Med 2010;44:555–62.
25. Junge A, Rosch D, Peterson L, et al. Prevention of soccer injuries: a prospective intervention study in youth amateur players. Am J Sports Med 2002;30:652–9.
26. McHugh MP. Oversized young athletes: a weighty concern. Br J Sports Med 2010; 44:45–9.

27. Nippert AH, Smith AM. Psychologic stress related to injury and impact on sports performance. Phys Med Rehabil Clin North Am 2008;19:399–418.

28. Biddle SJH, Asare M. Physical activity and mental health in children and adolescents: a review of reviews. Br J Sports Med, in press.

29. Smith AN, Link AA. Sport Psychology and the adolescent athlete. Pediatric Ann 2010;39:310–6.

30. Brenner JS; the Council on Sports Medicine and Fitness. Overuse injuries, overtraining, and burnout in child and adolescent athletes. Pediatrics 2007;119:1242–5.

31. Meeusen R, Nederhof E, Buyse L, et al. Diagnosing overtraining in athletes using the two-bout exercise protocol. Br J Sports Med 2010;44:642–8.

32. Bauman J. Returning to play: the mind does matter. Clin J Sports Med 2005;15: 432–5.

33. Brink MS, Visscher C, Arends S, et al. Monitoring stress and recovery: new insights for the prevention of injuries and illnesses in elite youth soccer players. Br J Sports Med 2010;44:809–15.

34. Micheli LJ. Should children be allowed to run marathon races? A virtual roundtable. Pediatr Exerc Sci 2006;18;1–10.

35. Micheli LJ, Glassman R, Klein M. The prevention of sports injuries in children. Clin Sports Med 2000;19;821–34.

36. Flynn JM, Lou JE, Ganley TL. Prevention of sports injuries in children. Curr Opin Pediatr 2002;14;719–22.

37. van Mechelen W, Hiobil H, Kemper HC. Incidence, severity, aetiology and prevention of sports injuries. A review of concepts. Sports Med 1992;14;82–99.

38. Emery CA. Risk factors for injury in child and adolescent sport: a systematic review of the literature. Clin J Sp Med 2003;13:256–68.

39. Micheli LJ. Overuse injuries in children's sports: the growth factor. Orthop Clin North Am 1983:14;337–60.

40. Micheli LJ, Curtis C. Stress fractures in the spine and sacrum. Clin Sports Med 2006;25:75–88.

Youth Sports Anterior Cruciate Ligament and Knee Injury Epidemiology: Who Is Getting Injured? In What Sports? When?

Kevin G. Shea, MD[a,b], Nathan L. Grimm, MD[a,b,*],
Christopher K. Ewing, DO[c], Stephen K. Aoki, MD[b]

KEYWORDS

• ACL • Knee Injury • Youth Sports • Epidemiology

The importance and benefits of exercise are well documented. With childhood obesity rates rising in most developed countries, encouraging outdoor play and sports participation may be one of several solutions for this problem. However, with the increased youth sport participation seen over the past 10 years, there has also been a need to monitor the risks of participation within this unique population. Unfortunately, only a few well-designed epidemiologic surveillance studies have been conducted thus far.

The pediatric and adolescent population is unique in that their skeletal system is still maturing, and thus, they may be susceptible to unique injury patterns and injury frequency. The frequency and severity of sports injuries can differ based on the type of exposure (competition vs practice), sport, gender, and age. Recording these variables is important to accurately determine risk and obtain reliable epidemiologic data. To do this, standard definitions for injury and exposure should be established and widely accepted.

Standardization of injury reporting will allow comparison of results across studies so the associated factors can be more thoroughly explored. The purpose of this article is to review the types and patterns of knee and anterior cruciate ligament (ACL) injuries for youth sports based upon recent research. Much of this review is based upon the extensive research of Comstock et al using data compiled from the National High School Sports-Related Injury Surveillance Study.[1] This article will focus on the

[a] Intermountain Orthopaedics, 600 North Robbins Road, Boise, ID 83702, USA
[b] University of Utah School of Medicine, Department of Orthopaedics, 590 Wakara Way, UT 84108, USA
[c] Western University of Health Sciences, 309 East 2nd Street, Pomona, CA 91766, USA
* Corresponding author.
E-mail address: ngrimm@intermountainortho.com

Clin Sports Med 30 (2011) 691–706
doi:10.1016/j.csm.2011.07.004
0278-5919/11/$ – see front matter © 2011 Elsevier Inc. All rights reserved.

high school–aged athlete, aged 14-18 years, as the data for this age group are more robust than the data for younger age groups. This report will focus on 9 major sports played at the high school level: boys' football, soccer, basketball, baseball, and wrestling and girls' soccer, basketball, volleyball, and softball.

REVIEW OF THE LITERATURE
Definitions

When referring to the data obtained from the National High School Sports-Related Injury Surveillance Study,[1] "injury" and "athletic-exposure" were defined as follows:

Injury[1]: (A) An injury that occurred as a result of participation in an organized high school competition or practice **and** (B) required medical attention by a team physician, certified athletic trainer, personal physician, or emergency department/urgent care facility **and** (C) resulted in restriction of the high school athlete's participation for one or more days beyond the day of injury **and** (D) any fracture, concussion, or dental injury regardless of whether or not it resulted in restriction of the student-athlete's participation.

Athletic exposure (AE)[1]: (A) One athlete participating in one practice or competition where he or she is exposed to the possibility of athletic injury.

Football (American)

Overview

In the United States, football remains one of the most popular sports with the largest number of high-school aged participants (over 1.1 million).[2] It also has one of the highest injury rates overall as well as the highest incidence of ACL injuries. Previous research reported the overall injury rates for football have been as high as 8.1 per 1000 exposures[3]; more recent data captured from a large nationwide surveillance study have shown a smaller but still relatively high rate of injury (3.81 overall, 12.96 competition, 2.06 practice[1]) (**Fig. 1**, **Table 1**). It is important to note that football has by far the highest injury rate per exposure during competition.

Injuries requiring surgery

Of the 9 sports studied, football has the second highest proportion of overall injuries that result in surgical intervention at 8.5% (**Table 2**).[1] In a recent unpublished study using the RIOS™ data, Allan et al reported that during the 2007-2009 seasons, football accounted for 69.5% of boys' ACL injuries and that approximately 60% of the ACL injuries recorded resulted in surgical intervention.[4]

Knee injury rates

The knee represents the second most common region injured during both competition (18.8%) and practice (13.6%) (**Tables 3–5**). Additionally, of the boys sports, football has the highest proportion of overall knee injuries than any other sport (16.5%).[1]

ACL injury rates

Overall, football has the second highest ACL injury rate (13.87 per 100,000 AEs) in the age group of 14-18 years old, ranking second to girls' soccer (14.08 per 100,000 AEs) (see **Fig. 1**) and has the fourth highest proportion of injuries with ACL etiology (3.64%) (**Fig. 2**).[5] Additionally, according to Allan et al's unpublished report, boys were 3 times more likely to sustain an ACL injury while playing football compared to any other sport discussed in this study.[4]

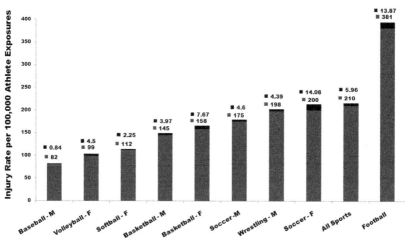

Fig. 1. Overall injury rate versus ACL injury rate per 100,000 athlete exposures by sport: High School Sports-Related Injury Surveillance Study, 2009–2010 school year. (An athlete exposure was defined as one athlete competing in one practice or competition.) (*Data from* the National High School Sports-Related Injury Surveillance Study, 2009–2010 School Year Summary: http://injuryresearch.net/resources/1/rio/2009-10HighSchoolRIOSummary/Report.pdf.)

Basketball

Overview
In the United States, it is estimated that more than 1 million high school–aged male and female athletes participate in basketball.[2] Comstock and colleagues' most recent

Table 1 Injury rates per 1000 athletic exposures* (Competition vs Practice) and sport: High School Sports-Related Injury Surveillance Study, 2009–2010 school year				
Sport	Competition Injury Rate*	Practice Injury Rate†	RR‡	P Value
All	4.19	1.32	3.17	<.001
Football	12.95	2.06	6.29	<.001
Soccer, boys	3.39	1.04	3.26	<.001
Soccer, girls	4.67	0.85	5.49	<.001
Volleyball, girls	1.00	0.99	1.01	.907
Basketball, boys	2.72	0.92	2.96	<.001
Basketball, girls	2.84	1.02	2.78	<.001
Wrestling, boys	3.09	1.56	1.98	<.001
Baseball, boys	1.27	0.57	2.23	<.001
Softball, girls	1.66	0.85	1.95	<.001

* A competition exposure was defined as one athlete participating in one competition.
† A practice exposure was defined as one athlete participating in one practice.
‡ Rate ratio = comparison of the competition injury rate to the practice injury rate.
Data from the National High School Sports-Related Injury Surveillance Study, 2009–2010 School Year Summary: http://injuryresearch.net/resources/1/rio/2009- 10HighSchoolRIOSummaryReport.pdf.

Table 2
Percent of injuries requiring surgery by sport and type of athletic exposure: high school sports related injury Surveillance Study, 2009–2010 school year

		Football (M)	Soccer (M)	Soccer (F)	Volleyball (F)	Basketball (M)	Basketball (F)	Wrestling (M)	Baseball (M)	Softball (F)
Percent of injuries requiring surgery by sport										
	All									
Total	8.0	8.5	7.6	8.4	6.4	9.0	7.2	6.5	8.0	6.4
Competition	9.3	9.7	9.7	9.2	13.6	9.7	9.1	10.3	5.8	4.9
Practice	6.3	7.0	5.0	6.4	3.2	8.2	4.6	3.2	11.0	7.6

M, male athletes; F, female athletes.

Data from the National High School Sports-Related Injury Surveillance Study, 2009–2010 School Year Summary: http://injuryresearch.net/resources/1/rio/2009-10High School RIOSummary Report.pdf.

Table 3
Most commonly injured body region by sport (overall)

Percent of All Injuries

	All	Football (M)	Soccer (M)	Soccer (F)	Volleyball (F)	Basketball (M)	Basketball (F)	Wrestling (M)	Baseball (M)	Softball (F)
Ankle	**17.5**	11.5	14.6	22.1	**38.9**	**33.6**	**41.2**	4.7	10.1	**17.4**
Head/face	**17.2**	**17.8**	**17.1**	**18.7**	13.1	**18.7**	**18.6**	**15.0**	**14.5**	**15.2**
Knee	**15.7**	**16.5**	11.9	**23.1**	**16.8**	**14.7**	**16.1**	11.8	9.0	10.0
Hand/wrist	10.3	12.0	9.1	4.4	6.2	9.1	6.0	7.5	**18.2**	**20.3**
Hip/thigh/upper leg	9.2	7.7	**19.8**	10.8	7.0	7.1	2.9	4.4	10.2	10.0
Shoulder	8.4	**12.7**	1.7	2.2	2.6	2.8	2.7	**15.1**	**13.7**	8.1
Trunk	5.8	6.0	6.6	6.3	6.5	3.5	3.5	9.4	3.6	6.1
Lower leg	4.7	4.3	7.4	6.5	4.6	2.2	1.7	3.7	5.3	4.3
Foot	4.1	3.4	7.9	3.8	3.8	6.4	4.8	1.5	4.2	2.8
Arm/elbow	4.0	3.8	3.5	1.3	0.2	1.6	1.0	**14.3**	11.4	5.1
Neck	1.9	2.4	0.3	0.7	0.0	0.1	0.0	11.8	0.0	0.7
Other	1.0	1.9	0.1	0.0	0.2	0.3	1.5	1.3	0.0	0.0

NOTE: M, male athletes; F, female athletes. Bolded categories indicate the top 3 injured anatomical locations for each sport.
Data from the National High School Sports-Related Injury Surveillance Study, 2009–2010 School Year Summary: http://injuryresearch.net/resources/1/rio/2009-10HighSchoolRIOSummaryReport.pdf.

Table 4
Most commonly injured body region by sport (competition)

	Percent of All Injuries										
	All	Football (M)	Soccer (M)	Soccer (F)	Volleyball (F)	Basketball (M)	Basketball (F)	Wrestling (M)	Baseball (M)	Softball (F)
Ankle	18.0	12.7	14.1	21.0	40.7	36.0	41.4	2.5	13.0	19.9
Head/face	21.1	20.3	27.5	20.6	17.7	21.0	21.6	18.0	21.4	18.2
Knee	17.8	18.8	11.2	24.0	24.2	16.9	17.1	11.1	11.0	13.1
Hand/wrist	9.0	11.0	4.6	5.2	9.2	9.3	3.2	4.1	19.3	17.0
Hip/thigh/upper leg	7.7	6.2	15.2	8.9	4.4	7.4	2.5	0.9	11.4	11.2
Shoulder	7.5	12.2	3.0	1.9	0.8	1.7	3.2	16.1	5.7	6.6
Trunk	5.5	5.4	7.3	6.1	0.0	2.4	5.5	12.6	2.2	4.3
Lower leg	4.3	4.1	8.4	6.3	0.6	0.5	0.3	3.7	3.6	3.5
Foot	2.7	2.1	4.8	3.7	2.4	2.9	3.5	1.1	0.0	3.7
Arm/elbow	4.3	4.5	3.4	1.6	0.0	1.3	1.7	17.2	12.3	2.6
Neck	1.8	2.4	0.5	0.7	0.0	0.0	0.0	12.3	0.0	0.0
Other	0.2	0.5	0.0	0.0	0.0	0.3	0.0	0.3	0.0	0.0

NOTE: M, male athletes; F, female athletes. Bolded categories indicate the top 3 injured anatomical locations for each sport.
Data from the National High School Sports-Related Injury Surveillance Study, 2009–2010 School Year Summary: http://injuryresearch.net/resources/1/rio/2009-10HighSchoolRIOSummaryReport.pdf.

Table 5
Most commonly injured body region by sport (practice)

Percent of All Injuries

	All	Football (M)	Soccer (M)	Soccer (F)	Volleyball (F)	Basketball (M)	Basketball (F)	Wrestling (M)	Baseball (M)	Softball (F)
Ankle	17	10	**15.2**	24.6	**38.1**	**30.7**	**40.9**	6.6	6.1	**15**
Head/face	**12.5**	**14.6**	4.5	14.1	**11**	**15.9**	**14.8**	**12.3**	5.3	**12.4**
Knee	**13.2**	**13.6**	12.9	20.9	**13.3**	**11.9**	**14.8**	11.4	6.2	7.3
Hand/wrist	12	13.3	**14.6**	2.4	4.8	8.9	9.5	10.6	**16.7**	**24.2**
Hip/thigh/upper leg	11	9.6	**25.3**	**15.6**	8.2	6.8	3.5	7.5	8.5	8.8
Shoulder	9.5	**13.4**	0.2	3	3.5	4.2	2	**14.2**	**28.5**	9.2
Trunk	6.2	6.8	5.6	6.6	9.5	4.7	1	6.6	1.2	7.6
Lower leg	5.1	4.5	6.1	7.2	6.4	4.2	3.5	3.7	7.6	4.9
Foot	5.9	5	11.6	4.2	4.5	10.6	6.5	1.9	9.7	2
Arm/elbow	4.3	3	3.6	0.6	0.3	1.9	0.2	**11.7**	**10.3**	7.2
Neck	1.8	2.5	0.1	0.8	0	0.2	0	11.4	0	1.3
Other	0.2	3.7	0.2	0	0.3	0.2	3.3	2.1	0	0

NOTE: M, male athletes; F, female athletes. Bolded categories indicate the top 3 injured anatomical locations for each sport.
Data from the National High School Sports-Related Injury Surveillance Study, 2009–2010 School Year Summary: http://injuryresearch.net/resources/1/rio/2009-10HighSchoolRIOSummaryReport.pdf.

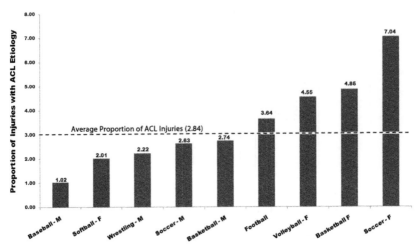

Fig. 2. Proportion of injuries with ACL etiology by sport: High School Sports-Related Injury Surveillance Study, 2009–2010 school year. (*Data from* the National High School Sports-Related Injury Surveillance Study, 2009–2010 School Year Summary: http://injuryresearch.net/resources/1/rio2009-10HighSchoolRIOSummaryReport.pdf.)

surveillance study indicated that basketball had the highest proportion of ankle injuries for both boys and girls (see **Tables 3–5**).[1] The task of determining the epidemiology of injury in young basketball athletes has been undertaken by several researchers looking at both local and regional samples[3,6–8] as well as samples taken nationwide.[9] Some of these studies have focused on identifying trends in injury rates relative to gender differences[10–12]; however, Comstock and colleagues surveillance study is the most robust surveillance study yielding these data.[1]

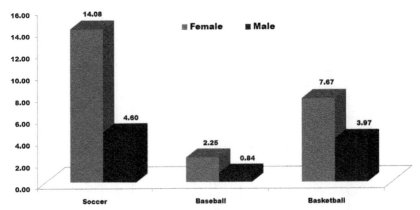

Fig. 3. ACL injury rate per 100,000 athlete exposures by sport and gender: High School Sports-Related Injury Surveillance Study, 2009–2010 school year. (An athlete exposure was defined as one athlete competing in one practice or competition.) (*Data from* the National High School Sports-Related Injury Surveillance Study, 2009–2010 School Year Summary: http://injuryresearch.net/resources/1/rio/2009-10HighSchoolRIOSummary/Report.pdf.)

Table 6

Rate ratio by gender and sport: High School Sports-Related Injury Surveillance Study, 2009–2010 school year

Rates of injury per 1000 athletic exposures and injury rate ratio by sport

	Soccer			Baseball/Softball			Basketball		
	Overall	Competition	Practice	Overall	Competition	Practice	Overall	Competition	Practice
Male athletes	1.75	3.39	1.04	0.82	1.27	0.57	1.45	2.72	0.92
Female athletes	**2.00**	**4.67**	0.85	**1.12**	**1.66**	**0.85**	**1.58**	**2.84**	**1.02**
RR* (95% CI)	1.14 (0.97–1.34)	1.38 (1.12–1.68)	1.23 (0.93–1.62)	1.36 (1.07–1.73)	1.30 (0.94–1.51)	1.47 (1.04–2.08)	1.09 (0.92–1.29)	1.04 (0.83–1.30)	1.11 (0.87–1.42)

* Rate ratio (RR) compares the gender with a higher injury rate (bolded) to the gender with a lower injury rate.

NOTE: All bolded values indicate a statistically significant difference between genders at 95% confidence interval not including 1.00.

Data from the National High School Sports-Related Injury Surveillance Study, 2009–2010 School Year Summary: http://injuryresearch.net/resources/1/rio/2009-10HighSchoolRIOSummaryReport.pdf.

Table 7 Most commonly injured knee structures for all sports: High School Sports-Related Injury Surveillance Study, 2009–2010 school year			
	Percent of All Injuries*		
Knee	Male Athletes	Female Athletes	Total
Medial collateral ligament	32.9	12.5	26.0
Anterior cruciate ligament	19.2	28.9	22.5
Patella and/or patellar tendon	18.1	29.1	21.8
Torn cartilage (meniscus)	20.0	15.8	18.6
Lateral collateral ligament	3.5	3.0	3.3
Post cruciate ligament	2.8	3.4	3.0

* Multiple responses per injury were allowed.
Data from the National High School Sports-Related Injury Surveillance Study, 2009–2010 School Year Summary: http://injuryresearch.net/resources/1/rio/2009-10HighSchoolRIOSummaryReport.pdf.

Injuries requiring surgery
In Borowski and colleagues' study,[9] although there was no statistically significant difference between the number of overall injuries requiring surgery when comparing boys to girls, there was a greater trend toward ligamentous sprain injuries requiring surgery in the female athletes.[9] However, there was a trend toward boys requiring more surgery for fracture care.[9]

Knee injury rates
Overall, knee injuries made up the third most common region injured for both boys (14.7%) and girls (16.1%). This was also true for boys and girls when stratifying by proportion of injuries occurring during competition (boys 19.9%, girls 17.1 %) and practice as well (boys 11.9%, girls 14.8%) (see **Tables 4** and **5**).

ACL injury rates
Among female athletes, basketball has the second highest incidence of ACL injuries next to soccer.[5] Girls' basketball also has the second highest proportion of ACL injuries and third highest overall injury rate among the sports, regardless of gender (4.85%) (see **Figs. 1** and **2**). For boys, soccer has a slightly higher ACL injury rate (4.60 per 100,000 AEs) than basketball (3.97 per 100,000 AEs)[5] (see **Fig. 1** and **Fig. 3**).

Gender differences
In 2008, Borowski et al published a comprehensive report on the epidemiology of basketball-related injuries using the data of the National High School Sports-Related Injury Surveillance Study,[13,14] which collected surveillance data from 100 randomly sampled high schools across the United States.[9] This study demonstrated that girls were more likely to experience a knee-related injury than were their male counterparts (P<.01). In this same study, injury rates among girls (1.58 overall, 2.84 competition, 1.02 practice) were slightly higher than those found in boys (1.45 overall, 2.72 competition, 0.92 practice) in all exposure environments.

Overall, for ACL injuries occurring in boy's basketball, the proportion of ACL injuries falls below the average when comparing them to the proportion of other sports played by the same gender (see **Fig. 2**). Conversely, for ACL injuries occurring in girl's basketball, the proportion of ACL injuries is above the average (see **Fig. 2**) and the injury rate remains marginally higher than boys (see **Fig. 3**).[5]

Soccer

Overview

With approximately 1 million high school–aged athletes participating in soccer nationwide[2] and countless other young athletes participating in club soccer year round, soccer has emerged as one of the most popular sports for both boys and girls. Due to soccer's restricted upper extremity use, with the exception of the goalie, there is a relatively low number of injuries seen in this region (**Tables 3–5**).[1] In contrast, however, the injury rate to the ACL is very high for both boys (4.06 per 100,000 AEs) and girls (14.08 per 100,000 AEs) (see **Figs. 1** and **3**).[5]

Injuries requiring surgery

A larger proportion of female soccer players sustained injuries requiring surgery compared with boys (8.4% girls, 7.6% boys) (see **Table 2**).[1] According to Allan et al's unpublished study, girls were twice as likely to sustain an ACL injury playing soccer than any other sport reviewed in his study and approximately 80% of ACL injuries required surgical intervention.[4]

Knee injury rates

For girls playing soccer, the knee is the most common site of injury (23.1%) whereas, for boys, the knee ranks as the forth most common site of injury (11.9%) (see **Table 3**).

ACL injury rates

Numerous studies have shown that girls are at a higher risk for ACL tears than boys and this risk appears to be between 2 to 3 times higher for girls.[15,16] Additionally, girls' soccer has the highest ACL injury rate for of all sports, whether boys' or girls'(14.08 or 100,000 AEs) (see **Fig. 1**). For boys, soccer has the second highest ACL injury rate (4.60 per 100,000 AEs)—second only to football.[5]

Gender differences

According to the National High School Sports-Related Injury Surveillance Study 2009-2010 data collected on young athletes,[1] boys had a lower overall injury rate (1.75 per 1000 AEs) than girls (2.00 injures per 1000 AEs).[1] Likewise, the rate of injury for boys in competition (3.39 injuries per 1000 AEs) was lower than for girls (4.67 injuries per 1000 AEs) in competition.[1] When considering injury location, girls appeared to be more likely to experience a soccer-related knee injury, whereas boys were more likely to experience a soccer-related injury to the hip/thigh/upper leg (see **Tables 3–5**).[1] In regard to ACL injuries, girls' soccer, basketball, and volleyball all had an above average proportion of ACL injuries when comparing all sports reviewed in this article (see **Fig. 2**).[5] Additionally, specific to soccer, both the injury rate for girls was 3 times as much as that for boys (see **Fig. 3**).[5]

A study reviewing insurance data for soccer athletes between the ages of 5 and 14 showed some interesting trends for youth ACL injuries.[17] This study had limitations because the number of injuries was recorded, but the number of athletes insured in specific age groups was not available. This study showed that ACL injury occurred at ages as young as 5 years in male athletes. Female athletes started sustaining ACL injury at higher rates around 12-14 years of age, and boys at around 14-16 years of age. Prior to these ages, ACL injuries were rare.[17] Throughout most age groups, the girls had a higher number of ACL injuries compared with boys. Although this study does have limitations, it is one of the few studies that included soccer athletes between the ages of 5 and 14.

Baseball/Softball

Overview

There are approximately a half million male high school athletes playing baseball,[2] 378 thousand female high school athletes playing softball,[2] and an estimated 6 million children playing organized baseball in the United States alone.[18] However, baseball and softball have the lowest ACL injury rates for their respective gender of the 9 major high school sports surveyed by Comstock and colleagues' summary report[5] (see **Fig. 1**).

Injuries requiring surgery

Of all injuries sustained by softball players during either competition or practice, 6.4% resulted in surgical intervention. For baseball players, this was slightly higher at 8.0%[1] (see **Table 2**). When the injuries were dichotomized into practice or competition, practice-related injuries required more surgery than injuries occurring during competition for both baseball (11.0%) and softball (7.6%), which was unique to these sports alone (see **Table 2**).

Knee injury rates

For both boys' baseball and girls' softball, knee injuries were not found to be in the top 3 most injured body regions for either competition or practice. More specifically, knee injuries were found to be the seventh most common site of injury for boys (9.0%) and the fourth most common sites of injury for girls (10.0%) (see **Table 3**).

ACL injury rates

Baseball injuries localized to the ACL occurred in 0.84 of 100,000 AEs for boys, whereas girls experienced 2.25 per 100,000 AEs.[5] Proportionally speaking, for baseball/softball, ACL injuries made up the smallest proportion of injuries compared to the other sports, making baseball and softball relatively low-risk sports for ACL injury (see **Figs. 1** and **2**).

Gender differences

The overall injury rate in both competition and practice is greater for girls playing softball than it is for their male counterparts playing baseball (**Table 6**).[1] For both boys playing baseball and girls playing softball, the largest proportion of injuries sustained during both competition and practice were of the sprain/strain type[1]; however, injuries to the knee were not found in the top 3 most common injuries (see **Tables 3–5**). Therefore, ACL injuries in these sports make up only a small fraction of the overall injury distribution. Nonetheless, girls still have a higher ACL injury rate when comparing the sports (see **Fig. 3**).

Volleyball

Overview

Volleyball is the third most popular sport played by high school–aged girls,[2] with more than 400,000 participants nationwide. Although volleyball is a 'noncontact' sport with opposing players separated by a net, this sport has the highest proportion of competition-related injuries requiring surgery compared to the other 8 sports reviewed here (see **Table 3**).[1] Previous studies have shown that ankle sprains are the most common injury,[19–24] and risk is increased when the player has experienced a previous ankle injury.[20–22] However, ACL injury rates among girls remains high in volleyball (4.50 per 100,000 AEs) despite being in the penultimate position for overall injury rates in the sports reviewed in this article (see **Fig. 1**).

Injuries requiring surgery
Of injuries occurring in practice, 3.6% required surgical management.[1] In contrast to this, 13.6% of injuries occurring during competition required surgery (see **Table 2**).[1] Of the 8 high school sports included in this surveillance study, this was the highest rate of competition-related injuries that required surgery.

Knee injury rates
Knee injuries are the second most common region injured during both competition (24.2%) and practice (13.3%) for girls' volleyball (see **Tables 4** and **5**).

ACL injury rates
The ACL injury rate for girls volleyball was found to be 4.50 per 100,000 AEs,[5] which makes it the third highest injury rate of the girls' sports reviewed (see **Fig. 1**). Interestingly, though, volleyball has the lowest number of overall injuries compared to other girls' sports (see **Fig. 1**).

Wrestling

Overview
Wrestling remains a very popular youth sport at the high school level, ranking sixth in the overall number of athletes enrolled.[2] Although the sport is known for its arduous nature and level of physical contact, the injury rate in high school–aged athletes is relatively low (3.09 of 1000 AEs in competition, 1.56 of 1000 AEs in practice),[1] with the proportion of ACL injuries being penultimate next to boys' basketball (see **Fig. 2**).

Injuries requiring surgery
Of injuries occurring during competition, 10.3% required surgery, whereas 3.2% of injuries during practice required surgery.[1] The aforementioned differences in proportion of injuries requiring surgery can be attributed to the degree of intensity during the different exposures.

Knee injury rates
Knee injuries were not found in the 3 most common regions injured but rather made up the sixth most common region injured during competition and the fourth most common region injured during practice (see **Tables 4** and **5**).

ACL injury rates
Although the injury rate of ACL injuries in wrestling is slightly less than that of boys' basketball, the injury rate is higher at 4.39 per 100,000 AEs.[5] However, when looking at the ACL injuries as a proportion of total injuries incurred, wrestling falls into the penultimate position for boys, and just slightly above softball (see **Fig. 1**).

DISCUSSION

Epidemiologic studies in sports medicine have played a vital role in identifying injury patterns within various sports. By analyzing epidemiologic data, we are able to provide recommendations to reduce the risk of injury for young athletes. Comprehensive data collection is the first step in identifying injury rates and athletes at risk. Further dissection of this data can then be used to recognize modifiable factors within sports including rule changes, implementing the use of protective equipment, limiting athlete exposure, and improving education and training programs. Specific examples of effective changes include pitch counts in youth baseball to minimize overuse injuries and banning "spear tackling" in American football to reduce cervical-spine injuries.[25,26]

Of particular importance in epidemiologic data is how we define an "injury." Standardizing definitions would allow comparisons among study populations. The current definition of "injury" as defined in The National High School Sports-Related Injury Surveillance Study by Comstock et al describes injuries in broad terms in order to maximize sensitivity of injury data collection. One of the most important aspects to collecting this type of data is identifying injuries that have the potential for long-term health effects. Future studies focusing on specific injuries are warranted with epidemiologic data guiding changes of modifiable factors. Clinically, it is also important to continue collecting data after rule changes to confirm that these changes are beneficial.

Current youth sports epidemiologic data has focused on injuries sustained at the high school level. Admittedly, some of these athletes have reached skeletal maturity and comprehensive epidemiologic data are currently limited to the late adolescent age group. Epidemiologic data in skeletally immature athletes are sparse; current literature is limited to surveillance data collected through coaches or emergency departments[27,28] or insurance data review.[17] Studies of this magnitude require comprehensive data collection, and current high school studies have relied heavily on the participation of certified athletic trainers (ATCs). ATCs have greatly enhanced the care of athletes and improved the timeliness of the medical evaluation, assessment, and treatment. The integral role ATCs play within high school sports has made it possible to observe and collect epidemiologic data and their role should not go unrecognized. Unfortunately, the use of ATCs in the pediatric setting (grade school, middle school, and club sports) is limited, and these data will be more challenging to collect. This is certainly a unique population and requires further evaluation.

SUMMARY

The study of knee and ACL injury is important, as these injuries may increase the risk of degenerative arthritis in the future. Of particular interest are the significantly higher rates of ACL injury seen in young female athletes. For this review, all 3 sports (baseball/softball, soccer, and basketball) demonstrated that female athletes have higher rates of ACL injury compared with male athletes. Some, but not all, recent studies have suggested that exercise prevention programs may reduce the risk of knee injury and ACL injury in these female athletes. Looking at the most commonly injured knee structures (**Table 7**), it is obvious that research in the field of prevention is needed. However, evaluation of the effectiveness of these intervention programs, as well as the age at which these programs should be implemented, requires further research.

REFERENCES

1. Comstock D, Collins CL, McIlvain NM. National High School Sports-Related Injury Surveillance Study. Summary Report 2010. Available at: http://www.injuryresearch.net/rioreports.aspx. Accessed February 1, 2011.
2. "2010–11 High-School Athletics Participation Survey". National Federation of State High School Associations. 2009–2010 High School Athletics Participation Survey. 2010. Available at: http://www.nfhs.org. Accessed February 1, 2011
3. Powell JW, Barber-Foss KD. McIlvain NM, et al. Injury patterns in selected high school sports: a review of the 1995–1997 seasons. J Athl Train 1999;34:277–84.
4. Allan JM, Yard E, McIlvain NM, et al. A multi-sport epidemiologic comparison of ACL injuries in high school athletics. Unpublished 2011.

5. Comstock D, Collins CL, McIlvain NM. High school sports-injury surveillance study. Unpublished raw data 2010. Available at: http://injuryresearch.net/rioreports.aspx. Accessed July 21, 2011.
6. Gomez E, DeLee JC, Farney WC. Incidence of injury in Texas girls' high school basketball. Am J Sports Med 1996;24:684–7.
7. Knowles SB, Marshall SW, Bowling JM, et al. A prospective study of injury incidence among North Carolina high school athletes. Am J Epidemiol 2006;164:1209–21.
8. Messina DF, Farney WC, DeLee JC. The incidence of injury in Texas high school basketball. A prospective study among male and female athletes. Am J Sports Med 1999;27:294–9.
9. Borowski LA, Yard EE, Fields SK, et al. The epidemiology of US high school basketball injuries, 2005-2007. Am J Sports Med 2008;36:2328–35.
10. Powell JW, Barber-Foss KD. Sex-related injury patterns among selected high school sports. Am J Sports Med 2000;28:385–91.
11. McKay GD, Goldie PA, Payne WR, et al. A prospective study of injuries in basketball: a total profile and comparison by gender and standard of competition. J Sci Med Sport 2001;4:196–211.
12. McQuillan R, Campbell H. Gender differences in adolescent injury characteristics: a population-based study of hospital A&E data. Public Health 2006;120:732–41.
13. Comstock D, Yard E, Knox CL, et al. National High School Sports-Related Injury Surveillance Study. Summary Report 2006. Available at: http://www.injuryresearch.net/rioreports.aspx. Accessed February 1, 2011.
14. Comstock D, Yard E, McIlvain NM. National High School Sports-Related Injury Surveillance Study. Summary Report 2007. Available at: http://www.injuryresearch.net/rioreports.aspx. Accessed February 1, 2011.
15. Walden M, Hagglund M, Werner J, et al. The epidemiology of anterior cruciate ligament injury in football (soccer): a review of the literature from a gender-related perspective. Knee Surg Sports Traumatol Arthrosc 2010.
16. Prodromos CC, Han Y, Rogowski J, et al. A meta-analysis of the incidence of anterior cruciate ligament tears as a function of gender, sport, and a knee injury-reduction regimen. Arthroscopy 2007;23:1320–5, e6.
17. Shea KG, Pfeiffer R, Wang JH, et al. Anterior cruciate ligament injury in pediatric and adolescent soccer players: an analysis of insurance data. J Pediatr Ortho 2004;24:623–8.
18. Kyle SB. Youth Baseball Protective Equipment Project. Final Report. Washington, DC: US Consumer Product Safety Commission; 1996.
19. Aagaard H, Scavenius M, Jorgensen U. An epidemiological analysis of the injury pattern in indoor and in beach volleyball. Int J Sports Med 1997;18:217–21.
20. Bahr R, Bahr IA. Incidence of acute volleyball injuries: a prospective cohort study of injury mechanisms and risk factors. Scand J Med Sci Sports 1997;7:166–71.
21. Bahr R, Karlsen R, Lian O, et al. Incidence and mechanisms of acute ankle inversion injuries in volleyball. A retrospective cohort study. Am J Sports Med 1994;22:595–600.
22. Verhagen EA, Van der Beek AJ, Bouter LM, et al. A one season prospective cohort study of volleyball injuries. Br J Sports Med 2004;38:477–81.
23. Watkins J, Green BN. Volleyball injuries: a survey of injuries of Scottish National League male players. Br J Sports Med 1992;26:135–7.
24. Schafle MD, Requa RK, Patton WL, et al. Injuries in the 1987 National Amateur Volleyball Tournament. Am J Sports Med 1990;18:624–31.
25. Boden BP, Tacchetti RL, Cantu RC, et al. Catastrophic cervical spine injuries in high school and college football players. Am J Sports Med 2006;34:1223–32.

26. Lyman S, Fleisig GS, Andrews JR, et al. Effect of pitch type, pitch count, and pitching mechanics on risk of elbow and shoulder pain in youth baseball pitchers. Am J Sports Med 2002;30:463–8.
27. Radelet MA, Lephart SM, Rubinstein EN, et al. Survey of the injury rate for children in community sports. Pediatrics 2002;110:e28.
28. Caine D, Maffulli N, Caine C. Epidemiology of injury in child and adolescent sports: injury rates, risk factors, and prevention. Clin Sports Med 2008;27:19–50, vii.

MR Imaging of ACL Injuries in Pediatric and Adolescent Patients

Victor M. Ho-Fung, MD*, Camilo Jaimes, MD,
Diego Jaramillo, MD, MPH

KEYWORDS
- Anterior cruciate ligament • Pediatric imaging
- Musculoskeletal • MRI • Trauma • Sports injuries

Magnetic resonance (MR) imaging of older children and adolescents who have suffered knee trauma has greatly improved the diagnostic evaluation of anterior cruciate ligament (ACL) tears and related injuries. Normal morphology, signal characteristics, and course of the ACL on MR images are well described in adults.[1,2] However, interpretation of diagnostic images in children requires a comprehensive understanding of normal development-related changes and injuries that are unique to the immature skeleton. This review focuses on the primary and secondary imaging findings of ACL injuries in the pediatric patient and describes the most significant development-related changes that occur in the knee throughout childhood.

TECHNICAL CONSIDERATIONS

MR imaging (MRI) is the main modality for visualization of the ACL. Injuries are shown best by a combination of high-resolution, high-signal-intensity images, and water-sensitive images. In the past, proton density (also called intermediate-weighted) images have provided high anatomic detail, and T2-weighted images and short Tau inversion recovery images have provided sensitivity to edema or fluid. Fat-saturated, intermediate-weighted sequences are increasingly used, because they have both high resolution and sufficient water sensitivity to detect edema. High resolution images require at least 120 to 140 mm field of view, matrices above 256 × 256, and a slice thickness of 3 mm or less. Our protocol includes an intermediate-weighted and a T2-weigthed sequence with fat suppression in the sagittal plane. The intermediate-weighted images depict the fibers of the ACL, and the T2-weighted images show edema in cases of ligamentous injuries as well as associated bone bruising.[3] In the coronal and axial planes, fat-saturated intermediate-weighted images usually suffice.

Department of Radiology, The Children's Hospital of Philadelphia, 34th & Civic Center Boulevard, 3NW 17, Philadelphia, PA 19104, USA
* Corresponding author.
E-mail address: hov@email.chop.edu

The authors prefer to include a series of T1-weighted images in the coronal plane, because they are more specific for marrow pathology and help distinguish a fracture from a bruise. The authors prefer also to make the axial image slightly T2 weighted to maintain anatomic resolution while detecting chondromalacia and other intrinsic cartilaginous abnormalities. In recent years, several authors have proposed imaging internal derangement of the knee with a single 3-dimensional (3D) sequence, based either on gradient recalled echo imaging[4] or fat-suppressed turbo spin intermediate-weighted imaging (**Fig. 1**).[5] 3T imaging, with a near 4-fold increase in signal to noise ratio, has proven to be adequate for evaluation of ACL pathology[6] and has greater sensitivity and specificity than 1.5T imaging for evaluation of cartilaginous defects in the knee.[7] However, there are greater magnetic susceptibility artifacts at 3T, and interference screws can produce significant distortion and hamper the evaluation of cartilage thickness.[8]

Normal Anatomy on MR Images

The normal ACL is an obliquely oriented band followed easily on midsagittal images, with its anterior border being straight and relatively parallel to Blumensaat's line (roof of the intercondylar notch).[1] It is of low signal intensity (SI) on all MR sequences, with a striated appearance, particularly at its femoral and tibial insertion sites, because of fat within its interstices. On axial images, it is most often seen on the first image in which the femoral cartilage becomes visible. On coronal images, its 2 functional bundles—the anteromedial and posterolateral—can be differentiated consistently. An oblique coronal image along the plane of the ACL can better separate the 2 bundles and help to detect subtle, incomplete tears. It is important to learn to follow the course of the ligament on all 3 planes to better confirm or discard a suspicion of a tear.

Development of the Knee

Although the presentation of skeletal injuries is related to the site of injury and the specific inciting event, in children it varies primarily with the degree of skeletal maturation. Awareness of development-related changes in the bone marrow, epiphyseal cartilage, and secondary ossification center, the physes, the menisci, and the ligaments of the knee is critical for the accurate diagnosis of injuries by MRI.[9]

The signal characteristics of the bones on MRI reflect the marrow composition.[9] In the neonate, for instance, all the marrow is hematopoietic and has low SI on T1-weighted images and high SI on water-sensitive sequences.[10] By the time skeletal maturity is reached, almost all the marrow in the appendicular skeleton is fatty, and thus has high SI on T1-weighted and low SI on water-sensitive sequences. In the extremities, marrow conversion from hematopoietic or red to fatty or yellow follows a predictable pattern from the periphery of the body (toes and fingers) toward the center (hips and shoulders).[11] Within each individual long bone, marrow transformation takes place in the epiphysis first, followed by the diaphysis and finally advancing toward the metaphyses. Thus, on T1-weighted images of a child's knee, the distal femoral and proximal tibial epiphysis have higher SI than the metaphyses, and typically the metaphysis of the distal femur will have more hematopoietic marrow than that of the proximal tibia (**Fig. 2**).[12]

At birth, the epiphyses of the long bones are primarily composed of hyaline cartilage and have a homogeneous intermediate SI on T1-weighted images and relatively low SI on water-sensitive sequences.[9] The cartilage of the primary physis has a higher SI than epiphyseal cartilage on all sequences. On water-sensitive sequences, the germinal and proliferative layers of the physis appear as a band of

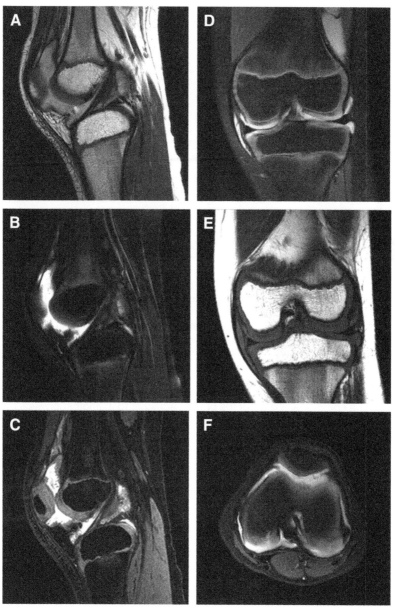

Fig. 1. Normal structure of the ACL in a 6-year-old girl. (*A*) Sagittal intermediate-weighted and (*B*) fat-saturated T2-weighted MR images of the knee show the normal course and SI of the ACL. A chronic knee effusion is also depicted. (*C*) Sagittal 3D gradient-recalled echo image shows the normal ACL and delineates the hyaline cartilage in the epiphyses of the distal femur, proximal tibia, and patella to a greater extent. (*D*) Coronal fat-saturated intermediate-weighted MR image shows the ACL at its tibial insertion. (*E*) Coronal T1-weighted MR image demonstrates the tibial insertion of the ACL, the femoral insertion of the PCL, and normal-appearing bone marrow in the metaphyses and epiphyses. (*F*) Axial fat-saturated intermediate-weighted MR image shows intact PCL, ACL, femoral cartilage, and patellar cartilage.

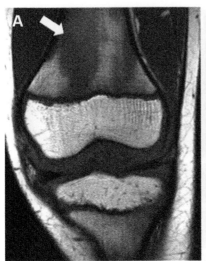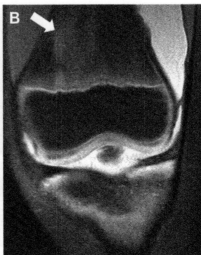

Fig. 2. Normal appearance of bone marrow in a 6-year-old girl with synovitis of the knee. (*A*) Coronal T1-weighted MR image of the knee demonstrates homogeneous high SI in the epiphysis of the distal femur and proximal tibia secondary to the presence of fatty marrow. Elongated, ill-defined foci of low SI representing residual red marrow in the metaphysis of the distal femur (*arrow*) are also seen. (*B*) Coronal fat-saturated intermediate-weighted MR image of the knee shows complete signal drop in the epiphysis and high SI in the metaphysis (*arrow*) owing to the higher water content of these foci of hematopoietic marrow. An effusion of the knee is also depicted.

high SI on the epiphyseal aspect of the physis. Adjacent to it, another physeal region, the zone of provisional calcification, can also be readily identified as a homogenously hypointense (dark) band on all pulse sequences (**Fig. 3**).[13]

In the child and adolescent, the epiphyseal cartilage of the distal femur has decreased SI along the weight-bearing region. Ossification changes in the posterior femoral condyles result in patches of high SI in the cartilage on T2-weighted images.[14] The secondary center of ossification is surrounded by a spherical secondary physis which has similar signal characteristics to the physis (**Fig. 4**).[9] During infancy and early childhood, the physes are gently arched and smooth. The physes of the distal femur and proximal tibia close centrally and this is seen as physeal undulation followed by loss of the bright signal from cartilage on MR images. The central physeal undulation is also the site of more complex physeal injuries and of secondary posttraumatic bony bridge formation.[15]

Trauma or orthopedic interventions can disrupt the physes around the knee[16] and create transphyseal bony bridges. The areas of bony bridging are seen as focal areas of decreased SI on T2-weighted images or gradient echo images. For instance, drill hole placement during ACL reconstruction produces a zone of low SI, which can be less than 5% of the physeal volume for both the femur and the tibia. The region of injury is peripheral, which carries a higher risk of physeal arrest.

Ligamentous and tendinous growth occurs as a consequence of bone lengthening[17] and there are changes in anatomic relationships between bones and ligaments at different ages. These changes have been well-documented in the knees of children on MRI. For instance, the site of insertion of the ACL in the tibia and the angle between the Blumensaat line and the ACL remain constant after 2 years of age. Conversely, the

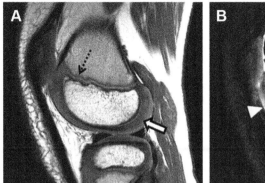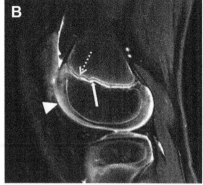

Fig. 3. Normal anatomy. (A) Sagittal intermediate-weighted MR image of the knee in a 6-year-old girl demonstrates the normal intermediate SI of the epiphyseal hyaline cartilage (*arrow*). A band of low SI corresponding to the zone of provisional calcification (*dotted arrows*) can be appreciated in the metaphyseal aspect of the growth plate in both images. (B) Sagittal, fat-saturated, T2-weighted MR image shows smooth bands of high SI in the distal femoral condyle (*thin arrow*) and around the secondary ossification center, corresponding with the primary and secondary physis, respectively. The articular cartilage (*arrowhead*) is clearly seen as a thin hyperintense rim surrounding the epiphyseal cartilage, which is of lower SI.

angles between the tibia and the ACL in the coronal and sagittal planes become progressively larger with advancing age, approaching adult standards after physeal closure (**Fig. 5**).[18] A similar age-related progression has been reported for the posterior cruciate ligament (PCL)–tibia angle, whereas the ratio of horizontal to vertical component of this ligament steadily decreases as subjects approach skeletal maturity (**Fig. 6**).[18]

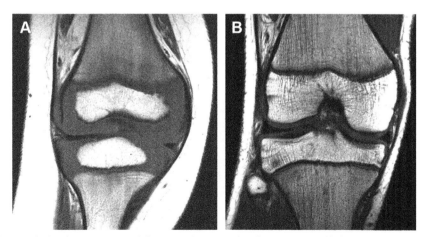

Fig. 4. Skeletal maturation. (A) Coronal T1-weighted MR image of the right knee in a 3-year-old boy shows cartilaginous epiphyses surrounding rounded secondary ossification centers in the distal femur and proximal tibia. (B) Coronal T1-weighted MR image of the knee in a 14-year-old boy demonstrates hemispheric ossification centers that conform to the contour of the primary physis of the distal femur, proximal tibia, and fibula.

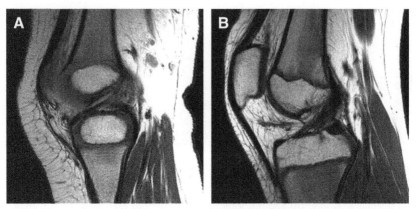

Fig. 5. Age-related changes in the ACL. Sagittal intermediate-weighted MR images of the knee in a (A) 2 year-old girl and (B) an 11 year-old girl show age-related increase in the ACL-tibia angle.

At birth, both menisci are highly cellular and vascular. Meniscal vascularity is seen on MR images as a line of high SI that bisects the meniscus horizontally, does not touch the articular surface, and extends to the meniscal attachment. Throughout childhood, the size of the menisci increases proportionally to the rest of the knee joint and the shape conforms to the articular surfaces of the tibia and femur. With age, there is a gradual decrease in the number of blood vessels, starting in the inner meniscal regions and progressing toward the periphery, so that by skeletal maturity the MR appearance of the meniscus resembles that of the adult.[19]

Determination of Skeletal Maturity

The management of patient's with skeletal injuries, especially in the case of ACL injuries requires accurate determination of the skeletal maturity in order to assess the

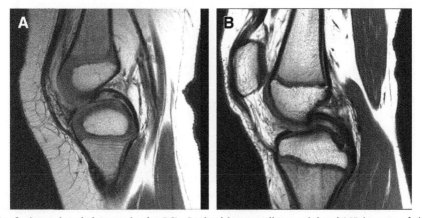

Fig. 6. Age-related changes in the PCL. Sagittal intermediate-weighted MR images of the knee in (A) a 2-year-old girl and (B) a 10 year-old girl show an increase in the PCL–tibia angle and a decrease in the quotient of horizontal to vertical component of the PCL.

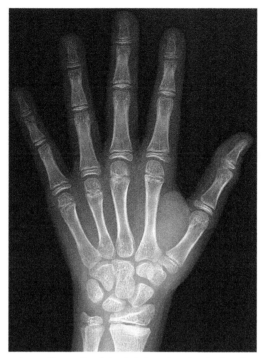

Fig. 7. Posterior anterior radiograph of the left hand and wrist in a boy with a chronologic age of 13 years and 1 month. Comparison with the Greulich and Pyle radiographic atlas of the hand and wrist revealed an apparent bone age of 13 years and 6 months with a standard deviation of 10 months. Because the bone age is within 2 standard deviations of the patient's chronologic age, the study was interpreted as normal.

amount of potential growth remaining.[20] Radiographic assessment of "bone age" in children older than 1 year uses a posteroanterior radiograph of the left hand and wrist to estimate physeal status and remaining growth (**Fig. 7**).[20,21] In general, assessment of the phalangeal epiphyses provides a more accurate evaluation of maturation than analysis of carpal and metacarpal bones. Comparison of the patient's bones with known standards is usually done using the Greulich and Pyle radiographic atlas of the hand and wrist. A normal bone age examination should be within 2 standard deviations from the mean chronologic age according to the Brush Foundation Study.[22] In the past decade, computer-based methods of evaluation of skeletal maturity have been developed and are currently being evaluated.

ACL INJURY

MRI is the preferred imaging modality for the diagnosis and assessment of ACL injuries. The overall sensitivity and specificity of MRI for the detection of ACL tears in children are 95% and 88%, respectively.[23] The sensitivity and specificity for individual primary findings of ACL tears have been reported to be 94% and 96% for abnormal angle with the Blumensaat line; 79% and 88% for increased SI in the substance of the ligament; and 21% and 100% for fiber discontinuity.[23]

ACL injury patterns vary substantially as a function of age. Avulsion fractures of the tibial eminence tend to occur during puberty, partial thickness tears in adolescents

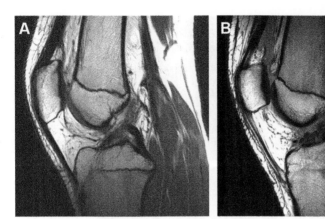

Fig. 8. (*A*) Sagittal intermediate-weighted MR image of the knee in a 14-year-old girl demonstrates abnormal signal in the substance of the ACL, which was interpreted as an incomplete tear. (*B*) Sagittal intermediate-weighted MR image of the knee in a different 14-year-old female who has a closed tibial physis shows discontinuity of the ACL fibers, consistent with a complete tear.

before skeletal maturity, and full-thickness tears after skeletal maturity (**Fig. 8**). In younger individuals with open physes, ACL injuries are more common in boys and frequently present as either tibial spine avulsions or incomplete tears. As skeletal maturation progresses, complete ligamentous tears are more commonly seen and affect females primarily.[24] Gender differences in morphology of the intercondylar notch, muscle strength, relative laxity of the ligaments, hormonal factors, and training differences are likely to account for these trends.[25]

Tibial Eminence Avulsion

In a child with an open or recently fused tibial physis, a sudden increase in the tension of the ACL may avulse the tibial eminence from the proximal tibial epiphysis. Radiographic evaluation of tibial eminence avulsion fractures should include frontal and lateral views of the knee. Determination of the degree of displacement of the fracture fragment is essential for application of the modified Meyers and McKeever classification.[26,27] This grading system describes a type I lesion as an avulsion fracture with minimal displacement from the proximal tibial physis, a type II lesion as a "hinged" type avulsion with displacement of one third to one half of the eminence with a persistent connection to the posterior portion of epiphysis, a type III lesion as a complete displacement of the fragment from its original attachment, and a type IV lesion as a comminuted fracture of the tibial eminence.[26]

Further characterization of the degree of displacement of the fragment in multiple planes and demonstration of associated injuries can be achieved using MRI (**Fig. 9**).[28,29] MRI depicts the avulsed fragment in association with a lax ACL. As with other avulsions, MRI shows relatively minor edema at the site of the bony separation. This is in contrast with impaction injuries, such as bone bruises, that result in significant and lasting marrow edema. Tibial eminence avulsions and midsubstance ACL injuries can coexist[30]; differentiating abnormal SI secondary to ligamentous retraction after an avulsion from a coexisting ACL tear can be challenging.

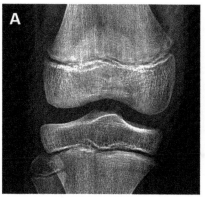
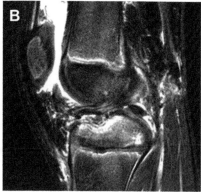

Fig. 9. (*A*) Anteroposterior radiograph of the knee in a 7-year-old boy shows a joint effusion and displacement of a fragment of the tibial eminence. (*B*) Sagittal, fat-saturated, T2-weighted MR image of the knee shows the avulsed fragment with associated high SI in the tibial epiphysis and in the midsubstance of the ACL.

Secondary Imaging Signs of ACL Injury

Because the ACL is the primary restraint of anterior tibial translation, about 72% of pediatric patients with deficient ACL's exhibit anterior tibial displacement.[24,31] MRI can document the ligamentous insufficiency (posterior-drawer equivalent) by demonstrating a posterior displacement of the femoral condyles relative to the margin of the tibia greater than 5 mm; the sensitivity and specificity of the latter finding for the diagnosis of ACL tears have been estimated to be 63% and 92%, respectively.[23] Uncovering of the posterior horn of the lateral meniscus is another associated finding, which occurs in approximately 18% of cases, has a sensitivity of 42%, and a specificity of 96%.[24,32] PCL buckling results from anterior translation of the tibia and is often assessed by measuring the angle between the femoral and tibial portions of the ligament. In children, this is an unreliable sign of ACL tear because the course of the PCL is more horizontal and the relationship between the horizontal and vertical components of the ligament changes with age.[33] Thus, a cutoff value set for adolescents will not work for young children. When using a cutoff value of 115°, the sensitivity and specificity of the PCL angle approach 74% and 71%, respectively, in the pediatric population.[23] A buckled PCL can be seen in the absence of a tear and may be exaggerated by hyperextension of the knee joint.[1,24,34]

Bone contusions are defined as subcortical areas of low SI on T1-weighted and high SI on T2-weighted or other water-sensitive images.[23] Patterns of bone contusion in the knee are helpful to identify the mechanism of injury.[35] The most common contusion pattern associated with ACL tears results from a pivot shift trauma and involves the lateral femoral condyle and posterolateral tibial plateau (**Fig. 10**).[24] Contusions in these locations have a sensitivity of 68% and a specificity of 88% for ACL tears.[23,36] The "deep lateral sulcus sign" is another pattern of bony contusion associated with ACL tears, which results from a subchondral impaction fracture along the lateral femoral condyle.[33,37]

Approximately 78% of ACL tears are associated with simple joint effusions. Although complex effusions are less common, they often occur as a result of injury to the ACL.[23] For instance, 47% of cases of acute knee hemarthrosis in children are associated with ACL tears.[24,38] Other complex effusions such as lipohemarthrosis suggest a marrow leak

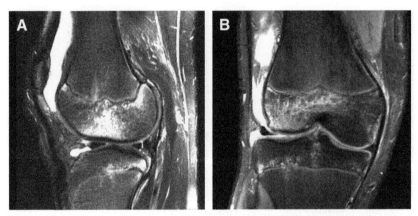

Fig. 10. A 15-year-old boy with an ACL tear and a joint effusion. (*A*) Sagittal, fat-saturated, T2-weighted and (*B*) coronal, fat-saturated, intermediate-weighted MR images demonstrate high SI corresponding with a bony contusion in the lateral femoral condyle and posterior aspect of the lateral tibial plateau.

and are concerning for a tibial eminence avulsion or a Salter–Harris fracture[25] (**Fig. 11**). In such cases, lipid material can be identified as a nondependent layer that follows the signal characteristics of fat on all pulse sequences.

IMAGING OF ACL GRAFT RECONSTRUCTION IN CHILDREN

Evaluation of the ACL graft can be performed with different imaging modalities. Radiographs allow assessment of tunnel positioning and integrity of the hardware. On the

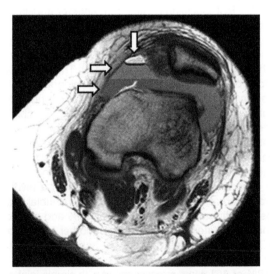

Fig. 11. A 15-year-old girl injured while playing basketball. Axial T1-weighted MR image shows a laterally displaced patella and a complex knee effusion with three distinct layers (*arrows*). The nondependent layer has a SI similar to that of subcutaneous fat, consistent with lipohemarthrosis.

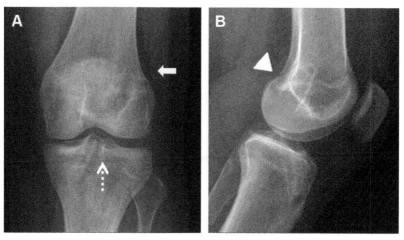

Fig. 12. A 14-year-old girl with a history of ACL tear and arthroscopic reconstruction using posterior tibial tendon allograft. (A) Frontal radiograph of the knee shows adequate orientation of the tunnel, with the femoral opening located above the lateral femoral condyle (*solid arrow*) and the tibial opening centered in the intercondylar eminence (*dotted arrow*). (B) Lateral radiograph of the knee better depicts the location of the posterior margin of the femoral tunnel at the intersection of the posterior cortex and the distal femoral physis (*arrowhead*).

frontal radiograph, the femoral tunnel should open above the lateral femoral condyle. The tunnel should be located between 10 and 11 o'clock on the right femur and 1 and 2 o'clock on the left femur. The graft should be angled less than 75° in the coronal plane to avoid graft laxity and maintain extension. On lateral radiographs, the posterior margin of the femoral tunnel should be at the intersection between the posterior cortex of the distal femur and the distal femoral physeal scar. The tibial tunnel should open at the intercondylar eminence; on lateral radiographs, its anterior margin should be directly posterior to a line along Blumensaat line intersecting the tibia (**Fig. 12**).[39]

In an attempt to reduce the risk of iatrogenic damage to the physis, several all epiphyseal ACL reconstruction techniques have been described.[40] One challenge is to create a tunnel through the epiphysis without harming the physis. At our institution, the all epiphyseal approach is performed using the O-arm intraoperative fluoroscopic unit for guidance. This provides a computed tomography data set that allows coronal and sagittal reconstructions of the physis and the epiphysis and maximal intensity projection images of these regions (**Fig. 13**).[40,41]

MRI can evaluate in more detail the integrity of the graft, hardware loosening, and possible complications such as ganglion cyst formation, graft impingement, iliotibial band friction syndrome, and arthrofibrosis.[42] An anterior position of the tibial tunnel can result in the graft being impinged by the roof of the intercondylar notch. With impingement, the graft shows increased SI, particularly in its anterior two thirds. The focal type of arthrofibrosis appears as a nodular soft tissue with heterogeneous low or intermediate SI in most MR sequences and is located immediately anterior to the distal end of the graft between the femur and the tibia. The diffuse form appears as a more extensive, ill-defined, soft tissue lesion within Hoffa's fat that surrounds the graft anteriorly and posteriorly. In addition, MRI can provide better assessment of joint fluid characteristics, synovial hypertrophy, intra-articular bodies, and meniscal and

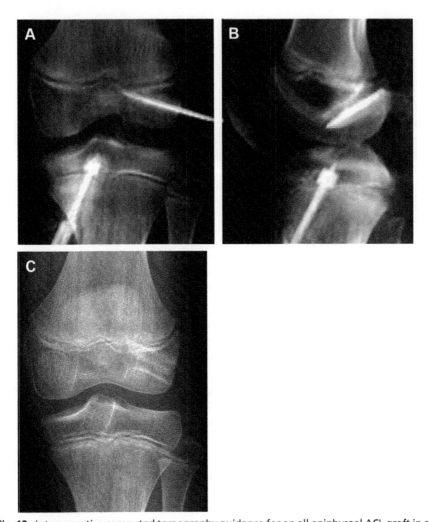

Fig. 13. Intraoperative computed tomography guidance for an all epiphyseal ACL graft in an 11-year-old boy with a complete ACL tear. (*A*) Coronal and (*B*) sagittal 3D reformations using maximum intensity projections demonstrate a femoral guide pin in the lateral femoral condyle in close proximity to the distal femoral physis, with the tip in the anatomic footprint of the ACL. The reconstructions also show drill hole with the tip at the tibial ACL footprint. (*C*) Frontal radiograph of the knee 4 months after the surgery shows the tunnels in both epiphyses. There is no evidence of physeal disruption.

articular chondral injuries. Particular attention should be given to early identification of bony bridges and possible angular deformities in skeletally immature patients after ACL graft reconstruction.[42]

CARTILAGE DEGENERATION AFTER ACL INJURIES

There are 2 main approaches to cartilage imaging: Morphologic and structural. In clinical practice, morphologic characterization of cartilage allows for identification of fractures, focal defects, and diffuse chondral processes, as well as anatomic evaluation after operative interventions. In children, imaging of cartilage should also allow for an adequate differentiation between zones of cartilage. Multiple sequences based on gradient recalled imaging and spin echo imaging can provide 3D maps of the cartilage and allow quantification of cartilage loss.[43]

To evaluate tissue composition, structural imaging of cartilage examines interactions between macromolecules in the extracellular matrix [collagen, proteoglycans, and (GAGs)], water, and mobile ions (sodium, Gd-DTPA^{-2}). T2-mapping is primarily influenced by the interaction (affinity) between water and collagen to identify changes in composition or hydration of the matrix. Degeneration of cartilage due to collagen breakdown results in longer T2 values. Imaging after ACL repair has shown higher T2 values in the tibiofemoral compartments, findings of deterioration of the integrity and orientation of the collagen network.[44]

Other techniques to evaluate the structural integrity of cartilage such as T (1ρ) and delayed gadolinium-enhanced MRI of cartilage reflect breakdown of GAGs. A study evaluating T(1ρ) values in the femoral and tibial cartilage in patients after ACL tear and reconstruction demonstrated persistent T(1ρ) signal abnormalities immediately after acute injuries and at the 1-year follow-up, primarily in the superficial layers of the cartilage.[45,46]

Delayed gadolinium-enhanced MRI of cartilage is based on the principle that anionic molecules such as those of Gd-DTPA^{-2} are normally repelled by the negative charges in the glycosaminoglycan molecules, but they can enter the cartilage where the glycosaminoglycan content decreases. The concentration of Gd-DTPA^{-2}, which varies inversely with the GAG content, can be measured by T1 mapping of cartilage. Sodium imaging measures sodium that naturally exist in cartilage to neutralize the anionic charges of GAGs; a decrease in the concentration of sodium directly reflects a decrease in the concentration of GAGs.[44] Together, these techniques provide information on tissue composition and allow a more accurate and prompt diagnosis of cartilage diseases.

KNEE INJURIES ASSOCIATED WITH ACL TEARS

When imaging the ACL, it is important to search for associated injuries. Certain MRI findings suggest specific mechanisms of injury that point to associated lesions. Overall, there seems to be a lesser incidence of associated injuries in younger children, perhaps because their musculoskeletal system is lighter and more compliant.[24]

The ACL and the medial meniscus are both restrictors of anterior tibial translation; therefore, once an ACL injury is detected, it is important to search carefully for an associated lesion in the medial meniscus.[24] Meniscocapsular separation associated with a posterior medial tibial plateau contusion can be seen as a result of a contrecoup injury during an ACL tear. The posterior horn of the medial meniscus should be tightly attached to the capsule, with no fluid in between the 2 structures. Separation is suggested when high SI fluid is seen in between the capsule and the medial meniscus. The meniscotibial fibers of the posterior oblique ligament are often also torn in this associated posteromedial corner injury. Alternatively, an ACL tear can coexist with a peripheral tear of the posterior horn of the medial meniscus.

In the pediatric population, MRI demonstrates meniscal injury with a sensitivity and specificity as high as 92% and 87%, respectively, for the medial meniscus and 93% and 95%, respectively, for the lateral.[47] On intermediate-weighted images, meniscal tears appear as areas of high SI that reach the articular surface of the meniscus. The menisci of children often have linear areas of high SI that correspond with meniscal vessels and should not be confused with tears.[28]

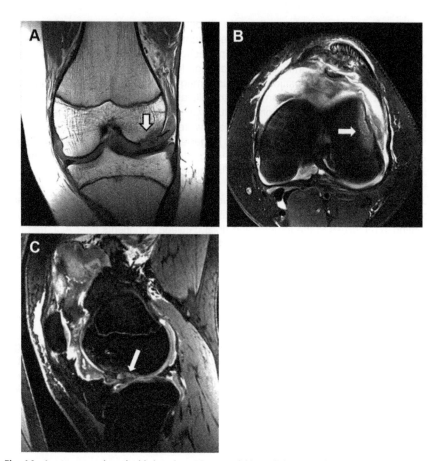

Fig. 14. Acute osteochondral injury in a 16-year-old boy. (*A*) Coronal T1-weighted MR image shows edema and a fracture of the articular cartilage of the lateral femoral condyle. (*B*) Axial intermediate-weighted MR image demonstrates a large complex joint effusion and edema of the subchondral bone. (*C*) Sagittal 3D gradient-recalled echo imaging delineates the articular cartilage and demonstrates a defect in the weight bearing portion of the lateral femoral condyle, suggesting an acute cartilage fracture.

ACL tears have been reported in 24% of patients with osteochondral injuries. Thus, the presence of the typical "kissing contusions," subchondral edema and impaction fractures should raise the concern for articular cartilage injury and prompt a dedicated assessment. MRI can detect a spectrum of abnormalities including thickening or blistering of the cartilage surface, superficial ulceration, deep fissuring, full-thickness chondral disruption with subchondral bone bruising and detachment of an osteo-chondral fragment (**Fig. 14**).[48] The Outerbridge classification can be used to describe MRI findings of these injuries.[49,50]

Discontinuity of the fibers of the medial collateral ligament is often see in association with tears of the ACL by the valgus stress component of pivot shift trauma. Combined injuries are seen 10 to 20 times more often in the medial than in the lateral collateral ligaments.[51] MR images show that the medial collateral ligament fibers are disrupted, and there may be associated injuries involving the medial

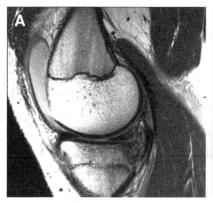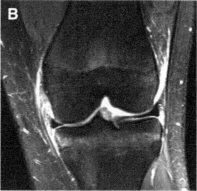

Fig. 15. A 13-year-old boy with a torn ACL. (*A*) Sagittal intermediate-weighted MR image of the knee shows increased SI and disruption of the posterior horn of the medial meniscus, consistent with a tear. (*B*) A coronal, fat-saturated, intermediate-weighted MR images of the knee show increased SI and discontinuity of the superior fibers of the medial collateral ligament, suggesting an associated tear.

meniscus (or meniscocapsular separation) and the ACL (O'Donoghue unhappy triad; **Fig. 15**).[52] There is increasing recognition that the lateral meniscus can also be torn, making this an even unhappier tetrad.[51] A partial ligamentous tear is seen as an area of increased SI within a thickened ligament. Complete tears are associated with more impressive soft tissue edema and a wavy configuration of the ligament with or without discontinuity of the fibers.[53]

Because the PCL is larger and stronger than the ACL, PCL tears are less frequent than those of the ACL and rarely occur simultaneously.[24,54] Sometimes on sagittal images, the meniscofemoral ligaments delineate the course of the absent PCL (**Fig. 16**). Although uncommon, avulsions of the tibial insertion of the PCL also have been described in children (**Fig. 17**).[55]

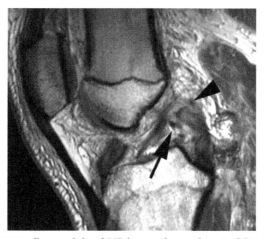

Fig. 16. Sagittal intermediate-weighted MR image shows abnormal SI and discontinuity of the PCL fibers, consistent with a tear. The anterior (*arrow*) and posterior (*arrowhead*) meniscofemoral ligaments are seen delineating the expected course of the PCL.

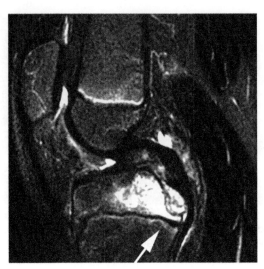

Fig. 17. Sagittal, fat-saturated, T2-weighted MR image shows an avulsion of the tibial PCL insertion (*arrow*) with associated high SI in the posterior aspect of the tibial epiphysis.

In patients with a PCL tear and a posterolateral corner complex,[56] severe instability may place an increased burden on the ACL. This may result in a primary tear of the ACL, or in failure of a previous ACL graft.[57] Different structures of the posterolateral corner of the knee, including the tendon of the biceps femoris, fibular collateral ligament, popliteus musculotendinous complex, fabellofibular ligament, and arcuate ligament, can be identified on MR images. Studies in adults have reported that instability is more likely to occur when 2 or more structures of the complex are injured,

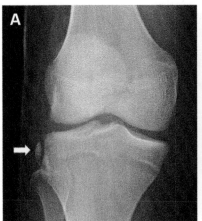
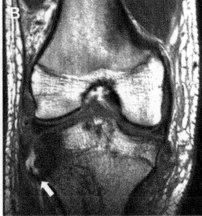

Fig. 18. Segond fracture in a 15-year-old boy. (*A*) Anterior posterior radiograph of the knee shows soft tissue edema and an avulsed bone fragment (*arrow*) in the lateral aspect of the knee. (*B*) Coronal T1-weighted MR image shows the displaced fragment accompanied by low SI bone marrow edema (*arrow*) in the tibia.

especially if the fibular collateral ligament, the popliteofibular complex or the postero-lateral joint capsule are involved.[58]

The Segond fracture, an avulsion fracture in the middle third of the lateral tibial rim,[59] can also be associated with an ACL tear. Radiographs of the knee usually demonstrate only a small avulsed fragment adjacent to the lateral tibial plateau, and MRI shows associated edema in the fracture bed and occasionally the avulsed fragment (**Fig. 18**).[59] MRI also demonstrates a much more significant ligamentous lesion. The injury usually involves complex mechanism of injury involving portions of the oblique band of the fibular collateral ligament and the iliotibial tract.[60] Even though Segond fractures are always considered to be strongly associated with ACL tears, recent studies in a pediatric population have reported them in fewer than 5% of ACL tears.[24]

SUMMARY

MRI is the preferred imaging modality for pediatric knee disorders such as tears of the ACL because it allows for accurate characterization of all the soft tissues in the joint without exposing the child to ionizing radiation. Imaging of the ACL is especially challenging and requires adequate understanding of the unique structural features of the pediatric skeleton, injury patterns as they relate to skeletal maturity and specific mechanisms of trauma.

REFERENCES

1. Roberts CC, Towers JD, Spangehl MJ, et al. Advanced MR imaging of the cruciate ligaments. Magn Reson Imaging Clin North Am 2007;15:73–86.
2. Moore SL. Imaging the anterior cruciate ligament. Orthop Clin North Am 2002;33:663–74.
3. Slattery T, Major N. Magnetic resonance imaging pitfalls and normal variations: the knee. Magn Reson Imaging Clin North Am 2010;18:675–89.
4. Duc SR, Pfirrmann CW, Koch PP, et al. Internal knee derangement assessed with 3-minute three-dimensional isovoxel true FISP MR sequence: preliminary study. Radiology 2008;246:526–35.
5. Kijowski R, Davis KW, Woods MA, et al. Knee joint: comprehensive assessment with 3D isotropic resolution fast spin-echo MR imaging—diagnostic performance compared with that of conventional MR imaging at 3.0 T. Radiology 2009;252:486–95.
6. Sampson MJ, Jackson MP, Moran CJ, et al. Three Tesla MRI for the diagnosis of meniscal and anterior cruciate ligament pathology: a comparison to arthroscopic findings. Clin Radiol 2008;63:1106–11.
7. Link TM, Sell CA, Masi JN, et al. 3.0 vs 1.5 T MRI in the detection of focal cartilage pathology—ROC analysis in an experimental model. Osteoarthritis Cartilage 2006;14:63–70.
8. Bowers ME, Tung GA, Trinh N, et al. Effects of ACL interference screws on articular cartilage volume and thickness measurements with 1.5 T and 3 T MRI. Osteoarthritis Cartilage 2008;16:572–8.
9. Laor T, Jaramillo D. MR imaging insights into skeletal maturation: what is normal? Radiology 2009;250:28–38.
10. Vogler JB 3rd, Murphy WA. Bone marrow imaging. Radiology 1988;168:679–93.
11. Burdiles A, Babyn PS. Pediatric bone marrow MR imaging. Magn Reson Imaging Clin North Am 2009;17:391–409.
12. Siegel MJ, Luker GG. Bone marrow imaging in children. Magn Reson Imaging Clin North Am 1996;4:771–96.

13. Khanna PC, Thapa MM. The growing skeleton: MR imaging appearances of developing cartilage. Magn Reson Imaging Clin North Am 2009;17:411–21.
14. Varich LJ, Laor T, Jaramillo D. Normal maturation of the distal femoral epiphyseal cartilage: age-related changes at MR imaging. Radiology 2000;214:705–9.
15. Ecklund K, Jaramillo D. Imaging of growth disturbance in children. Radiol Clin North Am 2001;39:823–41.
16. Shea KG, Apel PJ, Pfeiffer RP, et al. The anatomy of the proximal tibia in pediatric and adolescent patients: implications for ACL reconstruction and prevention of physeal arrest. Knee Surg Sports Traumatol Arthrosc 2007;15:320–7.
17. Connolly SA, Connolly LP, Jaramillo D. Imaging of sports injuries in children and adolescents. Radiol Clin North Am 2001;39:773–90.
18. Kim HK, Laor T, Shire NJ, et al. Anterior and posterior cruciate ligaments at different patient ages: MR imaging findings. Radiology 2008;247:826–35.
19. Clark CR, Ogden JA. Development of the menisci of the human knee joint. Morphological changes and their potential role in childhood meniscal injury. J Bone Joint Surg Am 1983;65:538–47.
20. Utukuri MM, Somayaji HS, Khanduja V, et al. Update on paediatric ACL injuries. Knee 2006;13:345–52.
21. Kirks DR, Griscom NT. Practical pediatric imaging: diagnostic radiology of infants and children. 3rd edition. Philadelphia: Lippincott-Raven; 1998.
22. Greulich WW, Pyle SI. Radiographic atlas of skeletal development of the hand and wrist. 2nd edition. Stanford (CA): Stanford University Press; 1959.
23. Lee K, Siegel MJ, Lau DM, et al. Anterior cruciate ligament tears: MR imaging-based diagnosis in a pediatric population. Radiology 1999;213:697–704.
24. Prince JS, Laor T, Bean JA. MRI of anterior cruciate ligament injuries and associated findings in the pediatric knee: changes with skeletal maturation. AJR Am J Roentgenol 2005;185:756–62.
25. Strouse PJ. MRI of the knee: key points in the pediatric population. Pediatr Radiol 2010;40:447–52.
26. Meyers AB, Laor T, Zbojniewicz AM. Stump entrapment of the anterior cruciate ligament in late childhood and adolescence. Pediatr Radiol 2011. [Epub ahead of print].
27. Zaricznyj B. Avulsion fracture of the tibial eminence: treatment by open reduction and pinning. J Bone Joint Surg Am 1977;59:1111–4.
28. Sanchez TRS, Jadhav SP, Swischuk LE. MR imaging of pediatric trauma. Magn Reson Imaging Clin North Am 2009;17:439–50.
29. Shea KG, Grimm NL, Laor T, et al. Bone bruises and meniscal tears on MRI in skeletally immature children with tibial eminence fractures. J Pediatr Orthop 2011;31:150–2.
30. Kocher MS, Mandiga R, Klingele K, et al. Anterior cruciate ligament injury versus tibial spine fracture in the skeletally immature knee: a comparison of skeletal maturation and notch width index. J Pediatr Orthop 2004;24:185–8.
31. Micheli LJ, Kocher MS. The pediatric and adolescent knee. Philadelphia: Saunders/Elsevier; 2006.
32. McCauley TR, Moses M, Kier R, et al. MR diagnosis of tears of anterior cruciate ligament of the knee: importance of ancillary findings. AJR Am J Roentgenol 1994;162:115–9.
33. Gentili A, Seeger LL, Yao L, et al. Anterior cruciate ligament tear: indirect signs at MR imaging. Radiology 1994;193:835–40.
34. Oeppen RS, Jaramillo D. Sports injuries in the young athlete. Top Magn Reson Imaging 2003;14:199–208.

35. Sanders TG, Medynski MA, Feller JF, et al. Bone contusion patterns of the knee at MR imaging: footprint of the mechanism of injury. Radiographics 2000;20(Spec No): S135–51.
36. Snearly WN, Kaplan PA, Dussault RG. Lateral-compartment bone contusions in adolescents with intact anterior cruciate ligaments. Radiology 1996;198:205–8.
37. Cobby MJ, Schweitzer ME, Resnick D. The deep lateral femoral notch: an indirect sign of a torn anterior cruciate ligament. Radiology 1992;184:855–8.
38. Stanitski CL, Harvell JC, Fu F. Observations on acute knee hemarthrosis in children and adolescents. J Pediatr Orthop 1993;13:506–10.
39. Zbojniewicz A. Postoperative imaging in adolescents with a focus on the knee. In: Morrison BFA, Jaramillo D, Kielar A, editor. Imaging of the Active Life Style From the weekend warrior to the Pro Athlete. Leesburg (VA): American Roentgen Ray Society; 2011. p.171–5.
40. Lawrence JT, Bowers AL, Belding J, et al. All-epiphyseal anterior cruciate ligament reconstruction in skeletally immature patients. Clin Orthop Relat Res 2010;468: 1971–7.
41. Gupta R, Cheung AC, Bartling SH, et al. Flat-panel volume CT: fundamental principles, technology, and applications. Radiographics 2008;28:2009–22.
42. Bencardino JT, Beltran J, Feldman MI, et al. MR imaging of complications of anterior cruciate ligament graft reconstruction. Radiographics 2009;29:2115–26.
43. Jaramillo D. Cartilage imaging. Pediatr Radiol 2008;38(Suppl 2):S256–8.
44. Crema MD, Roemer FW, Marra MD, et al. Articular cartilage in the knee: current MR imaging techniques and applications in clinical practice and research. Radiographics 2011;31:37–61.
45. Theologis AA, Kuo D, Cheng J, et al. Evaluation of bone bruises and associated cartilage in anterior cruciate ligament-injured and -reconstructed knees using quantitative t(1rho) magnetic resonance imaging: 1-year cohort study. Arthroscopy 2011; 27:65–76.
46. Li X, Kuo D, Theologis A, et al. Cartilage in anterior cruciate ligament-reconstructed knees: MR imaging T1{rho} and T2—initial experience with 1-year follow-up. Radiology 2011;258:505–14.
47. Major NM, Beard LN Jr, Helms CA. Accuracy of MR imaging of the knee in adolescents. AJR Am J Roentgenol 2003;180:17–9.
48. Oeppen RS, Connolly SA, Bencardino JT, et al. Acute injury of the articular cartilage and subchondral bone: a common but unrecognized lesion in the immature knee. AJR Am J Roentgenol 2004;182:111–7.
49. Outerbridge RE. The etiology of chondromalacia patellae. J Bone Joint Surg Br 1961;43-B:752–7.
50. Potter HG, Linklater JM, Allen AA, et al. Magnetic resonance imaging of articular cartilage in the knee. An evaluation with use of fast-spin-echo imaging. J Bone Joint Surg Am 1998;80:1276–84.
51. Palmer WE. Magnetic resonance imaging of knee trauma: biomechanical approach. Top Magn Reson Imaging 2003;14:161–78.
52. O'Donoghue DH. The unhappy triad: etiology, diagnosis and treatment. Am J Orthop 1964;6:242–7.
53. Al-Otaibi L, Siegel MJ. The pediatric knee. Magn Reson Imaging Clin North Am 1998;6:643–60.
54. Kennedy JC, Hawkins RJ, Willis RB, et al. Tension studies of human knee ligaments. Yield point, ultimate failure, and disruption of the cruciate and tibial collateral ligaments. J Bone Joint Surg Am 1976;58:350–5.

55. Ugutmen E, Sener N, Eren A, et al. Avulsion fracture of the posterior cruciate ligament at the tibial insertion in a child: a case report. Knee Surg Sports Traumatol Arthrosc 2006;14:340–2.
56. Fanelli GC, Edson CJ. Posterior cruciate ligament injuries in trauma patients: part II. Arthroscopy. 1995;11:526–9.
57. LaPrade RF, Resig S, Wentorf F, et al. The effects of grade III posterolateral knee complex injuries on anterior cruciate ligament graft force. A biomechanical analysis. Am J Sports Med 1999;27:469–75.
58. Vinson EN, Major NM, Helms CA. The posterolateral corner of the knee. AJR Am J Roentgenol 2008;190:449–58.
59. Gottsegen CJ, Eyer BA, White EA, et al. Avulsion fractures of the knee: imaging findings and clinical significance. Radiographics 2008;28:1755–70.
60. Campos JC, Chung CB, Lektrakul N, et al. Pathogenesis of the Segond fracture: anatomic and MR imaging evidence of an iliotibial tract or anterior oblique band avulsion. Radiology 2001;219:381–6.

Tibial Eminence Fractures

Christian N. Anderson, MD[a], Allen F. Anderson, MD[b],*

KEYWORDS
- Tibial spine • Tibial eminence • ACL avulsion • Pediatric

Tibial eminence fracture, a bony avulsion of the anterior cruciate ligament (ACL) from its insertion on the intercondylar eminence,[1] was first described by Poncet in 1875.[2] Also known as tibial spine fractures, these injuries occur most commonly in skeletally immature patients between the ages of 8 and 14 years.[3] They account for 2% to 5% of knee injuries in the pediatric population[4,5] and 14% of ACL injuries,[6] and have an incidence of 3 per 100,000 children per year.[7] Although tibial eminence fractures are relatively rare, pediatric knee injuries, in general, are increasing in frequency secondary to increased competitive sports participation,[8,9] and present a public health problem because of the detrimental effects they can have on the health and well-being of young athletes.[10] Given these concerns, appropriate treatment of tibial eminence fractures is paramount to the restoration of knee function, return-to-sports participation, and overall quality of life.

ANATOMY

The tibial intercondylar eminence is an elevated region of bone between the medial and lateral tibial condyles. It is anatomically divided into 4 distinct regions—a medial and lateral intercondylar spine and an anterior and posterior recess[11,12]—and serves as an insertion point for the cruciate ligaments and menisci.[12,13] The ACL is oriented obliquely, originating from the posteromedial side of the lateral femoral condyle, and inserting into a broad oval- or triangular-shaped region in the medial portion of the anterior recess.[12–15] The anterior fibers of the ACL flatten out anteriorly and blend with the insertional fibers of the anterior horn of the medial meniscus, whereas the posterior ACL fibers insert into the base of the medial spine and blend with anterior insertion of the anterior horn of the lateral meniscus.[13,14,16]

MECHANISM

In the pediatric population, tibial eminence fractures are most likely to occur while children are participating in various sports, eg, falling from a bike and skiing.[17–19] The

The authors have nothing to disclose.
[a] Department of Orthopaedic Surgery, Vanderbilt University Medical Center, 1215 21st Avenue South, Suite 4200, Medical Center East, South Tower, Nashville, TN 37232, USA
[b] Tennessee Orthopaedic Alliance/The Lipscomb Clinic, Suite 1000 Street Thomas Medical Building, 4230 Harding Road, Nashville, TN 37205, USA
* Corresponding author.
E-mail address: andersonaf@toa.com

Clin Sports Med 30 (2011) 727–742
doi:10.1016/j.csm.2011.06.007
0278-5919/11/$ – see front matter © 2011 Published by Elsevier Inc.

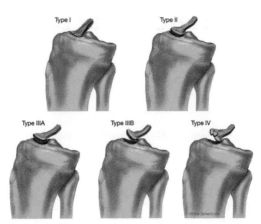

Fig. 1. Classification system of tibial eminence fractures. Type I, nondisplaced or minimally displaced anterior margin; type II, the anterior 1/3 to 1/2 of the fragment is displaced; type IIIA, complete displacement of the fragment; type IIIB, complete displacement and cephalad rotation of the fragment; type IV, comminution of the fragment. (*Courtesy of* Delilah Cohn, MFA, CMI, Nashville, TN.)

mechanism of injury is similar to intrasubstance ACL tears—hyperextension of the knee with a valgus or rotational force.[3,20–23] In a biomechanical study on primates, Noyes and colleagues[1] found that eminence fractures are more likely to occur at slower loading rates compared with intrasubstance ACL tears. In children, the weakness of their incompletely ossified tibial plateau relative to the ACL results in an avulsion fracture as tensile load is applied.[3,23] Before bone failure, an in situ stretch injury of the ACL may occur[1] and may result in clinical laxity despite adequate reduction of the fracture fragment.[24–26]

CLASSIFICATION

ACL avulsion fractures may vary considerably in the size of fragment, depth of the fracture into the tibial plateau, degree of displacement, and amount of comminution.[27] These injuries may also result in complete or incomplete ACL avulsions, with the majority of incomplete avulsions involving the anteromedial bundle.[27] The most commonly used classification system is based on 4 fracture patterns that vary in degrees of displacement and comminution (**Fig. 1**). Meyers and McKeever[28] defined types I to III. A type I fracture is the least severe, with a nondisplaced or minimally displaced anterior margin and excellent bony apposition. In a type II fracture, the anterior 1/3 to 1/2 of the fragment is displaced, with an intact posterior hinge. Type III fractures are classified in 2 subcategories. Type IIIA avulsion fractures have complete separation of the fragment from the bony bed without apposition, and type IIIB fractures are completely displaced and rotated cephalad. Zaricznyi[29] described type IV fractures, which represent comminution of the fragment.

DIAGNOSIS

A patient with a tibial eminence fracture typically presents with a painful knee hemarthrosis, decreased range of motion, and difficulty bearing weight.[24] Physical examination should include a complete neurologic and vascular examination of the lower extremity, as well as a thorough musculoskeletal examination of the knee.

Several studies have shown an association between eminence fractures and injury to the collateral ligaments, menisci, and articular cartilage.[30–32] Surgeons should be cognizant of these associated injures and treat them appropriately when encountered.

Radiographic evaluation should include anteroposterior (AP) and lateral radiographs of the knee, the latter of which is particularly useful in determining the degree of displacement of the fracture fragment. Although radiographs are used to make the diagnosis, in skeletally immature patients the fracture fragments may be considerably larger than how they appear on radiograph, because a significant part of the fragment may be cartilaginous.[23] Computed tomographic scanning allows improved visualization of the fracture fragment compared with radiographs and provides a more precise assessment of the fracture and presence of comminution.[27] Magnetic resonance imaging (MRI) can be helpful in preoperative planning by identifying concomitant injuries of the knee and the position of the fragment relative to the soft tissue structures that may impede reduction.[19,33,34] MRI is also useful in determining if interstitial injury of the ACL is present.[19]

TREATMENT

Tibial eminence fractures vary significantly in regards to fracture type, associated intraarticular injury, entrapment of soft tissue within the fracture site, and extension of fracture into the tibial plateau.[18,23,27,35] Treatment is based on these characteristics and tailored to each fracture pattern. Displaced tibial eminence fractures disrupt the continuity of the femur-ACL-tibial viscoelastic chain and can cause mechanical block to knee extension. The goals of treatment, therefore, are to restore continuity of the ACL and its stabilizing function, eliminate the mechanical block caused by the fragments, and restore congruity of the tibial plateau.[27,35–37]

TYPE I FRACTURE

The general consensus among researchers is that type I fractures can be treated nonoperatively with long-leg cast immobilization.[6,22,23,26,28,38–44] Aspiration of the knee hemarthrosis may be performed before casting to decrease swelling and pain. Although there is agreement on treatment with immobilization among researchers, opinions on knee position during treatment vary. McLennan[45] demonstrated in cadavers and in vivo that greatest tension of the ACL occurred at 0° and 45° of flexion, whereas the least tension was noted at 30° of flexion. Some researchers immobilize the knees in "slight flexion,"[23, 41] whereas others recommend immobilization at specific knee flexion angles. Meyers and McKeever[46] and Willis and colleagues[38] recommended placing the knee in 20° of flexion, Beaty and Kumar[43] recommended 10° to 15° of flexion, and Fyfe and Jackson[42] immobilized knees at 30° to 50° of flexion.

Although most investigators treat type I fractures with immobilization in flexion, others place the knee in full extension[22,41] or hyperextension.[26] However, placing the knee in hyperextension may cause discomfort for the patient[23] and can theoretically increase the risk of compartment syndrome because of excessive tension on the popliteal artery.[3] Even so, Wilfinger and coworkers[19] treated 14 skeletally immature patients with type I fractures with aspiration and closed reduction in hyperextension for 3 weeks, followed by conversion to a cast with 10° to 15° of knee flexion. In this series, no compartment syndromes or complaints of discomfort were reported.

Healing occurs rapidly in skeletally immature patients, and most researchers have treated type I fractures with 4 to 6 weeks of immobilization.[6,19,22,38] Radiographs should be obtained immediately after casting to ensure maintenance of fracture reduction and weekly or bimonthly thereafter. The duration of immobilization depends on the patient's age, signs of radiographic union, and the patient's compliance and motivation. To prevent the stiffness associated with immobilization of tibial spine fractures, the shortest period of immobilization possible is recommended.[23,35,40]

TYPE II FRACTURE

The treatment of type II fractures is more controversial than that of type I fractures; both operative and nonoperative treatments have been recommended. Nonoperative treatment typically involves cast immobilization for 4 to 6 weeks, with or without aspiration, and closed reduction of the knee in extension.[19,41] Wiley and Baxter[23] showed that the fracture line can extend into the tibial plateau, which supports the use of closed reduction to allow the femoral condyles to hold the fragment reduced. However, in a cadaveric study, McLennan[45] showed that the footprint of the femoral condyle was not congruous with the fracture line at any point of flexion. Even so, some investigators have hypothesized that extension causes the fat pad to act as a space-occupying cushion that holds the fracture reduced regardless of its size.[47] Meyers and McKeever,[46] in contrast, warned that closed reduction may convert a type II fracture to a type III fracture. If closed reduction is attempted, fluoroscopy should be used to confirm adequate position of the fragment, and the patient should be followed up closely to confirm maintenance of reduction in the cast. Kocher and colleagues[18] were only successful in closed reduction in 26 of 49 patients with type II fractures. Of those fractures that were irreducible, 26% were found to have soft tissue entrapment within the fracture preventing reduction.[18] Senekovic and Veselko[48] found intermeniscal ligament entrapment in 5 of 8 type II fractures. If an acceptable fracture reduction cannot be achieved by closed manipulation or if concurrent intraarticular injuries are present, operative treatment is indicated.

TYPE III/IV FRACTURES

Closed reduction and immobilization can be attempted in type III or IV tibial spine fractures (**Fig. 2**A). This technique is less successful in maintaining fracture reduction because the fragment is completely displaced.[39,41,45,49] The lower likelihood of success with closed reduction may be due, in part, to the higher incidence of soft tissue entrapment observed in this fracture pattern.[18,48] Kocher and coworkers[18] found 65% and Senekovic and Veselko[48] found 100% of type III fractures had intermeniscal ligament, anterior horn of medial meniscus, or anterior horn of the lateral meniscus incarcerated within the fracture. However, Lowe and colleagues[49] found no tissue interposition in 12 type III fractures, but they observed that extension of the knee caused displacement of the fracture fragment by pulling the anterior horn of the lateral meniscus that inserted on the osteochondral fragment. Given the difficulties associated with nonoperative management, most authors have recommended operative fixation for type III or IV fractures. Operative treatment regimens have included open reduction with casting,[39,41] open reduction with internal fixation (ORIF),[6,23,38,39] arthroscopic reduction with casting,[38,46] and arthroscopic reduction and internal fixation (ARIF) with sutures,[20,32,36,50–65] metal screws,[22,25,31,48,66–68] bioabsorbable nails,[69] Kirschner wires,[23,30,38,39] and, more recently, suture anchors.[70–73]

The best ARIF technique has not yet been determined because of the paucity of comparative studies in the literature. In a cohort study, Seon and coworkers[37] compared suture with screw fixation in type II and type III fractures and found no difference in functional outcomes. Biomechanical studies to determine the fixation

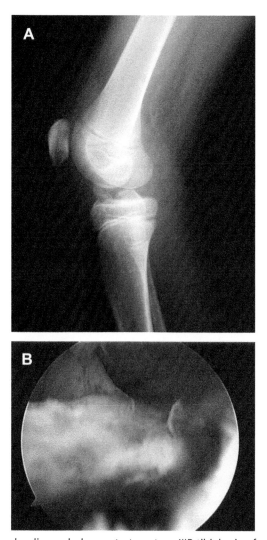

Fig. 2. (*A*) This lateral radiograph demonstrates a type IIIB tibial spine fracture in a 12-year-old male. (*B*) This arthroscopic view shows the type IIIB tibial spine fracture after the entrapped intermeniscal ligament was retracted with a 2-0 Prolene suture.

strength of various techniques have had mixed results.[74–77] In a porcine model, Eggers and colleagues[75] demonstrated that FiberWire sutures (Arthrex, Naples, FL, USA) were superior to Ethibond sutures (Ethicon, Norderstedt, Germany) and 1 or 2 antegrade cannulated screws in both cyclic and single-cycle loading protocols. They found that the use of 2 cannulated screws weakens the bone fragment, resulting in earlier failure.[75] Bong and coworkers[77] also found that FiberWire sutures were significantly stronger than 1 cannulated screw in a single-cycle failure test. In a bovine model, Mahar and colleagues[74] found no difference between Ethibond suture, bioabsorbable nails, a single bioabsorbable screw, or a single metal screw in an ultimate failure test. In a cyclical loading test, Tsukada and coworkers[76] found a statistically significant difference in displacement favoring an antegrade cannulated screw over Ethibond sutures.

Comminuted fractures should be treated with suture fixation, because screws are unlikely to provide adequate fixation.[6,60] With screw fixation, the fracture fragment should be at least 3 times the size of the screw diameter[60] to prevent disruption of the fragment. However, a second surgery may be needed for hardware removal if the screw head is prominent.[78]

SURGICAL TECHNIQUE

In the recent literature, ARIF, rather than open surgery, has become the standard of care. A mini-arthrotomy for ORIF may still be necessary in fractures that are irreducible by arthroscopic means.[37] In skeletally immature patients, physeal sparing techniques should be used to prevent growth disturbance.[79] The following techniques are based on our previous work.[80]

Setup

The operative extremity is placed in a circumferential leg holder with the hip flexed to 20° to allow lateral fluoroscopic imaging of the knee. A tourniquet is used to reduce bleeding and improve visualization. The C-arm is placed on the opposite side of the injured leg, and the tibial physis is visualized in the AP and lateral planes before the limb is prepped and draped.

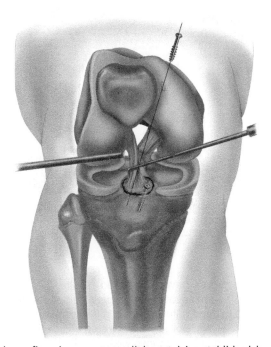

Fig. 3. With the knee flexed, a superomedial portal is established by first inserting an 18-gauge spinal needle at the level of the mid to upper patella at an angle that is as perpendicular as possible to the tibial plateau. A portal is established at this location. After the fracture fragment is reduced, a 1.25-mm threaded A-0 guide wire is inserted into the fragment, the hole is drilled with C-arm visualization, and the appropriate 3.5-mm self-tapping cannulated cancellous screw is inserted.

Screw Fixation

Standard anterolateral and anteromedial portals are created and the knee is lavaged to remove the hemarthrosis. A systematic examination is performed and any meniscal pathology should be treated at this time. A shaver is then used to resect the ligamentum mucosum and enough of the infrapatellar fat pad to allow adequate visualization. The fracture fragment is elevated, and residual blood clot and debris are removed with a shaver or small curette (**Fig. 2**B). With the knee in 60° of flexion, a superomedial portal is established at the level of the mid to upper patella by first inserting an 18-gauge spinal needle as perpendicular as possible relative to the tibial plateau. Soft tissue incarcerated in the fracture crater can be retracted with a probe through this portal. If the tissue cannot be retracted with the probe, a suture may be placed through the anteromedial portal into the soft tissue and used to extract the soft tissue from the fracture. A probe or Freer elevator is used through the anteromedial

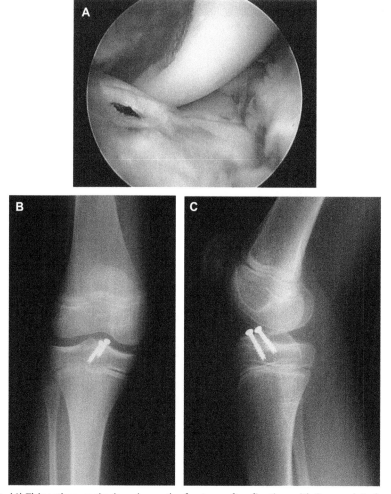

Fig. 4. (*A*) This arthroscopic view shows the fracture after fixation with 2 cannulated screws. (*B, C*) The corresponding radiograph demonstrates reduction of the fragment.

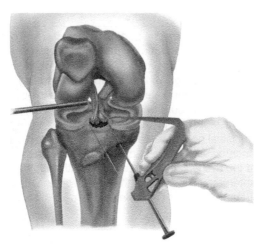

Fig. 5. An ACL drill guide, inserted through the anteromedial portal, is used to insert two 2.4-mm drill-tip guide pins that enter the joint at the lateral and medial edges of the fracture crater.

portal to reduce the fragment. A 1.25-mm thread-tip guide wire is inserted through the superomedial portal under real-time fluoroscopy into the anterior medial half of the fragment. The guide wire should be stopped before entering the tibial physis. Carefully insert the guide wire as perpendicular to the fracture as possible. A second

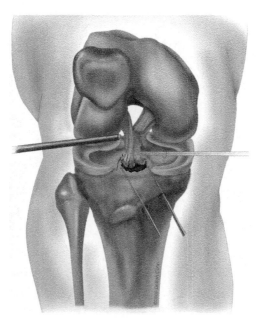

Fig. 6. A Spectrum suture passer is used to pass a 2-0 Prolene suture or shuttle relay through the posterior fibers of the ACL.

guide wire can be placed into the anterolateral half of the fragment to serve as provisional fixation while the screw is being inserted. A cannulated measuring device is placed over the guide wire, and a partially threaded, cannulated screw of appropriate length is selected. The wire is then overdrilled with a 2.7-mm cannulated drill bit under fluoroscopy, again avoiding the physis. The self-tapping 3.5-mm screw is then inserted. A second screw can be placed over the provisional guide wire if the fragment is large enough (**Fig. 3**). The knee is extended to determine if the screw head impinges on the femur (**Fig. 4A, B, C**). A small notchplasty may be performed if necessary to prevent impingement.

Suture Fixation

The initial preparation for arthroscopic suture fixation is similar to that for screw fixation. The fracture is reduced, and a thread-tip, 1.25-mm guide wire is inserted into the anterior central portion of the fragment for provisional fixation. For Tanner stage I, II, or III patients, the physis may be avoided by using a transepiphyseal rather than a transphyseal technique. Using C-arm visualization, an ACL drill guide is introduced through the anteromedial portal. Determine the entrance site of the pins on the anteromedial aspect of the tibia epiphysis by advancing the drill sleeve to the skin. A 2-cm to 3-cm incision is made in this location and the periosteum is elevated. The ACL drill guide and a 2.4-mm drill-tip guide wire are used to make 2 parallel tunnels 1 cm apart that enter at the medial and lateral edges of the fracture crater on either side of the ACL insertion (**Fig. 5**). The drill guide is removed, and a Spectrum suture passer (Conmed Linvatec, Largo, FL, USA) with a 90° tip is used to pass a 2-0 Prolene suture through the posterior fibers of the ACL as close to the bony fragment as possible (**Fig. 6**). Both ends of the suture are then retrieved with a grasper through a 5-mm cannula in the anteromedial portal. The suture is used to shuttle a #2 FiberWire (Arthrex) through the ACL (**Fig. 7**).

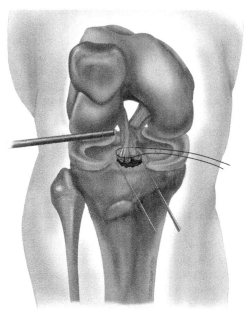

Fig. 7. A #2 FiberWire is shuttled through the ACL and pulled out the medial portal.

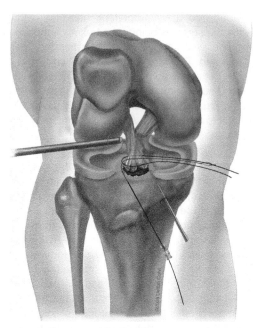

Fig. 8. The lateral guide pin is removed first and an 18-gauge spinal needle is placed in the drill hole. A CHIA suture passer is inserted through the spinal needle and is pulled out through the medial portal. The FiberWire suture limb on the medial side of the ACL is then loaded on the CHIA suture passer and pulled out through the lateral tibial drill hole.

The lateral pin is removed first and replaced with an 18-gauge spinal needle. A CHIA suture passer (Depuy Mitek, Raynham, MA, USA) is inserted through the spinal needle into the knee and retrieved through the cannula in the medial portal. The medial limb of the FiberWire suture is loaded on the CHIA passer and pulled through the lateral drill hole (**Fig. 8**). The lateral limb of the FiberWire suture is passed through the medial drill hole in a similar manner, creating a loop around the anterior portion of the ACL (**Fig. 9**). A second #2 FiberWire is passed through the base of the ACL more anterior than the first. The limbs are passed in the same manner as before, and the sutures are tied independently over the 1-cm bone bridge on the anteromedial tibial epiphysis (**Fig. 10**).

Postoperative Regimen

Place the patient in a long-leg, hinged-knee brace that is locked in extension. Encourage the patient to do quadriceps muscle contractions and straight leg raises. The day after the surgery, initiate range-of-motion exercises (ROM) and hamstring stretching in the prone position. Toe-touch weight-bearing with crutches is allowed. Progression to full weight-bearing can begin 6 weeks after surgery. Active ROM exercises, including terminal extension, and patella mobilization can also begin 6 weeks after surgery. Exercises are introduced in levels of increasing difficulty. Patients can resume participating in sports within 4 to 6 months of surgery.

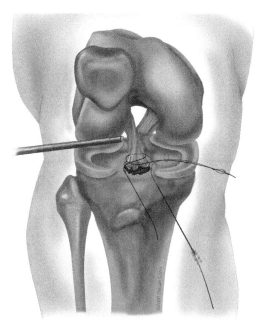

Fig. 9. The medial drill-tip guide pin is then removed and, using the same technique, the lateral FiberWire suture limb is passed out through the medial hole creating a loop around the ACL and the fracture fragments.

DISCUSSION

Despite generally good results, complications of both operative and nonoperative treatments may occur in children with tibial spine fractures, including residual laxity, loss of motion, nonunion, and growth deformity.

Residual laxity is one of the most common complications and has been reported with both operative[24,25] and nonoperative[19,39,40] treatment of all fracture patterns. Anterior laxity may be due, in part, to interstitial elongation of the ACL at the time of injury[1] and/or soft tissue interposition that impedes fracture reduction.[18] Despite the presence of objective residual laxity, many researchers found that most patients have no complaints of instability.[23,24,38,40] Residual laxity may be asymptomatic because preservation of proprioceptive feedback allows normal neuromuscular control of the knee.[22] However, other studies report that increased laxity associated with interstitial elongation results in worse outcomes.[26,45] McLennan[45] reviewed a series of type III fractures treated with closed reduction and immobilization (CRI), arthroscopic reduction and immobilization (ARI), and ARIF. He reported that International Knee Documentation Committee (IKDC), Lysholm, and Tegner scores were highest in those undergoing ARIF and lowest in the CRI group.[45] Anterior laxity was lowest in ARIF and highest in CRI. Second-look arthroscopy revealed fracture displacement in CRI and ARI groups, and 6 of 7 patients treated with immobilization had retropatellar chondromalacia.[45] Although most authors recommend an anatomic reduction,[17,18,24,48] others recommend countersinking the fragment to account for interstitial injury and minimize residual laxity.[25,72]

Loss of motion, a common problem after treatment of tibial spine fractures, may be caused by arthrofibrosis or malunion of the fracture. Arthrofibrosis has been attributed

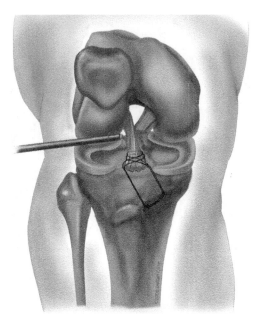

Fig. 10. A second suture is then passed through the ACL fibers more anterior than the first and the limbs are passed through the same tibial drill holes as described.

to prolonged postoperative immobilization.[23,35,40,81] The use of rigid internal fixation may allow more aggressive rehabilitation in an attempt to minimize stiffness.[81] Fracture malunion may occur as a result of incomplete reduction during nonoperative treatment[45] or malreduction during operative treatment of displaced fractures.[68] Femoral notchplasty has been used to regain extension in cases of malunion.[82,83]

Nonunion, although uncommon, has been associated with nonoperative treatment of displaced fractures.[55,56] Zhao and Huangfu[55] presented a series of nonunions of type II and III fractures that were treated with removal of the fibrous tissue and ARIF using sutures. This treatment restored normal laxity in 10 of 11 patients. The IKDC scores in these patients improved from abnormal or severely abnormal to normal or nearly normal.[55]

Iatrogenic growth disturbance, an uncommon complication after fixation of tibial spine fractures, may cause significant impairment. Mylle and colleagues[79] presented a case report of an 11-year-old girl treated with a transphyseal screw for a displaced tibial eminence fracture. Hardware was left in place for 2 years postoperatively. The patient had premature closure of the anterior half of the growth plate, resulting in 25° hyperextension, 30° loss of flexion, and instability during sports.[78] Ahn and Yoo[56] reported a series of displaced fractures treated with absorbable suture fixation through the tibial physis, with 2 cases of growth deformity. Given the potential severity of iatrogenic growth disturbance, physeal sparing techniques are recommended to fix tibial eminence fractures in skeletally immature patients.[56,63,79]

ACKNOWLEDGMENTS

The authors thank Tracey Fine of Fine Biomedical Publications, Inc for editing the manuscript.

REFERENCES

1. Noyes F, DeLucas J, Torvik P. Biomechanics of anterior cruciate ligament failure: an analysis of strain-rate sensitivity and mechanisms of failure in primates. J Bone Joint Surg Am 1974;56(2):236–53.
2. Poncet A. Arrachement de l'epine du tibia a l'insertion du ligament croise anterieur. Bull Mem Soc Chir Paris 1875;1:883–4.
3. Zionts L. Fractures and Dislocations about the Knee. In: Green NE, Swiontkowski MR, editors. Skeletal trauma in children. Philadelphia: WB Saunders; 2009. p. 452–5.
4. Luhmann S. Acute traumatic knee effusions in children and adolscents. J Pediatr Orthop 2003;23:199–202.
5. Eiskjaer S. The significance of hemarthrosis of the knee in children. Arch Orthop Trauma Surg 1988;107(2):96–8.
6. Kendall N, Hsy S, Chan K. Fracture of the tibial spine in adults and children. A review of 31 cases. J Bone Joint Surg Br 1992;74(6):848–52.
7. Skak S, Jensen TT, Poulsen TD, et al. Epidemiology of knee injuries in children. Acta Orthop Scand 1987;58:78–81.
8. Anderson A. Transepiphyseal replacement of the anterior cruciate ligament in skeletally immature patients: a preliminary report. J Bone Joint Surg Am 2003;85-A(7): 1255–63.
9. Stanitski C, Harvell J, Fu F. Observations on acute knee hemarthrosis in children and adolescents. J Pediatr Orthop 1993;13(4):506–10.
10. Yang J. Use of discretionary protective equipment and rate of lower extremity injury in high school athletes. Am J Epidemiol 2005;161(6):511–9.
11. Agur A. Grant's atlas of anatomy. 9th edition. Baltimore: Williams and Wilkins; 1991.
12. Clemente C. Anatomy: a regional atlas of the human body. 4th edition. Baltimore: Williams and Wilkins; 1997. p. 387–8.
13. Girgis F. The cruciate ligaments of the knee joint. Anatomical, functional and experimental analysis. Clin Orthop Relat Res 1975;(106):216–31.
14. Petersen W. Anatomy of the anterior cruciate ligament with regard to its two bundles. Clin Orthop Relat Res 2007;454:35–47.
15. Harner C. Quantitative analysis of human cruciate ligament insertions. Arthroscopy 1999;15(7):741–9.
16. Messner K. The menisci of the knee joint. Anatomical and functional characteristics, and a rationale for clinical treatment. J Anat 1998;193(Pt 2):161–78.
17. Casalonga A, Bourelle S, Chalencon F, et al. Tibial intercondylar eminence fractures in children: the long-term perspective. Orthop Traumatol Surg Res 2010;96:525–30.
18. Kocher M, Micheli LJ, Gerbino P, et al. Tibial eminence fractures in children: prevalence of meniscal entrapment. Am J Sports Med 2003;31(3):404–7.
19. Wilfinger C, Castellani C, Raith J, et al. Nonoperative treatment of tibial spine fractures in children-38 patients with a minimum follow-up of 1 year. J Orthop Trauma 2009;23(7):519–24.
20. Lubowitz J. Part II: arthroscopic treatment of tibial plateau fractures: intercondylar eminence avulsion fractures. Arthroscopy 2005;21(1):86–92.
21. Accousti W. Tibial eminence fractures. Orthop Clin North Am 2003;34(3):365–75.
22. Ahmad C, Stein BE, Jeshuran W, et al. Anterior cruciate ligament function after tibial eminence fracture in skeletally mature patients. Am J Sports Med 2001;29(3):339–45.
23. Wiley J, Baxter M. Tibial spine fractures in children. Clin Orthop Relat Res 1990;(255): 54–60.
24. Perugia D. Clinical and radiological results of arthroscopically treated tibial spine fractures in childhood. Int Orthop 2009;33(1):243–8.

25. Kocher M, Foreman E, Micheli L. Laxity and functional outcome after arthroscopic reduction and internal fixation of displaced tibial spine fractures in children. Arthroscopy 2003;19(10):1085–90.
26. Tudisco C. Intercondylar eminence avulsion fracture in children: long-term follow-up of 14 cases at the end of skeletal growth. J Pediatr Orthop B 2010;19(5):403–8.
27. Griffith J, Antonio GE, Tong CW, et al. Cruciate ligament avulsion fractures. Arthroscopy 2004;20(8):803–12.
28. Meyers M, McKeever F. Fracture of the intercondylar eminence of the tibia. J Bone Joint Surg Am 1959;41-A(2):209–20[discussion: 220–2].
29. Zaricznyi B. Avulsion fracture of the tibial eminence: treatment by open reduction and pinning. J Bone Joint Surg Am 1977;59(8):1111–4.
30. McLennan J. The role of arthroscopic surgery in the treatment of fractures of the intercondylar eminence of the tibia. J Bone Joint Surg Br 1982;64(4):477–80.
31. Binnet M, Gürkan I, Yilmaz C, et al. Arthroscopic fixation of intercondylar eminence fractures using a 4-portal technique. Arthroscopy 2001;17(5):450–60.
32. Montgomery K, Cavanaugh J, Cohen S, et al. Motion complications after arthroscopic repair of anterior cruciate ligament avulsion fractures in the adult. Arthroscopy 2002;18(2):171–6.
33. Toye L, Cummings P, and Armendariz G. Adult tibial intercondylar eminence fracture: evaluation with MR imaging. Skeletal Radiol 2002;31(1):46–8.
34. Prince J, Laor T, Bean J. MRI of anterior cruciate ligament injuries and associated findings in the pediatric knee: changes with skeletal maturation. AJR Am J Roentgenol 2005;185(3):756–62.
35. Hunter R, Willis J. Arthroscopic fixation of avulsion fractures of the tibial eminence: technique and outcome. Arthroscopy 2004;20(2):113–21.
36. Medler R, Jansson K. Arthroscopic treatment of fractures of the tibial spine. Arthroscopy 1994;10(3):292–5.
37. Seon J, Park SJ, Lee KB, et al. A clinical comparison of screw and suture fixation of anterior cruciate ligament tibial avulsion fractures. Am J Sports Med 2009;37(12):2334–9.
38. Willis R, Blokker C, Stoll TM, et al. Long-term follow-up of anterior tibial eminence fractures. J Pediatr Orthop 1993;13(3):361–4.
39. Janarv P, Westblad P, Johansson C, et al. Long-term follow-up of anterior tibial spine fractures in children. J Pediatr Orthop 1995;15(1):63–8.
40. Baxter M, Wiley J. Fractures of the tibial spine in children. An evaluation of knee stability. J Bone Joint Surg Br 1988;70(2):228–30.
41. Molander M, Wallin G, Wikstad I. Fracture of the intercondylar eminence of the tibia: a review of 35 patients. J Bone Joint Surg Br 1981;63-B(1):89–91.
42. Fyfe I, Jackson J. Tibial intercondylar fractures in children: a review of the classification and the treatment of mal-union. Injury 1981;13(2):165–9.
43. Beaty J, Kumar A. Fractures about the knee in children. J Bone Joint Surg Am 1994;76(12):1870–80.
44. Lileros K, Werner S, Janarv P. Arthroscopic fixation of anterior tibial spine fractures with bioabsorable nails in skeletally immature patients. Am J Sports Med 2009;37(5):923–8.
45. McLennan J. Lessons learned after second-look arthroscopy in type III fractures of the tibial spine. J Pediatr Orthop 1995;15(1):59–62.
46. Meyers M, McKeever F. Fracture of the intercondylar eminence of the tibia. J Bone Joint Surg Am 1970;52(8):1677–84.
47. Ogden John A. Skeletal injury in the child. 3rd edition. New York: Springer-Verlag: 2000. p. 1001.

48. Senekovic V, Veselko M. Anterograde arthroscopic fixation of avulsion fractures of the tibial eminence with a cannulated screw: five-year results. Arthroscopy 2003;19(1): 54–61.
49. Lowe J, Chaimsky G, Freedman A, et al. The anatomy of tibial eminence fractures: arthroscopic observations following failed closed reduction. J Bone Joint Surg Am 2002;84-A(11):1933–8.
50. Kim Y, Kim SJ, Yang JY, et al. Pullout reattachment of tibial avulsion fractures of the anterior cruciate ligament: a firm, effective suture-tying method using a tensioner. Knee Surg Sports Traumatol Arthrosc 2007;15(7):847–50.
51. Kogan M, Marks P, Amendola A. Technique for arthroscopic suture fixation of displaced tibial intercondylar eminence fractures. Arthroscopy 1997;13(3):301–6.
52. Lehman R, Murphy KP, Machen MS, et al. Modified arthroscopic suture fixation of a displaced tibial eminence fracture. Arthroscopy 2003;19(2):E6.
53. Jung Y, Yum J, Koo B. A new method for arthroscopic treatment of tibial eminence fractures with eyed Steinmann pins. Arthroscopy 1999;15(6):672–5.
54. Delcogliano A, Chiossi S, Caporaso A, et al. Tibial intercondylar eminence fractures in adults: arthroscopic treatment. Knee Surg Sports Traumatol Arthrosc 2003;11(4): 255–9.
55. Zhao J, Huangfu X. Arthroscopic treatment of nonunited anterior cruciate ligament tibial avulsion fracture with figure-of-8 suture fixation technique. Arthroscopy 2007; 23(4):405–10.
56. Ahn J, Yoo J. Clinical outcome of arthroscopic reduction and suture for displaced acute and chronic tibial spine fractures. Knee Surg Sports Traumatol Arthrosc 2005;13(2):116–21.
57. Yang S, Lu YC, Teng HP, et al. Arthroscopic reduction and suture fixation of displaced tibial intercondylar eminence fractures in adults. Arch Orthop Trauma Surg 2005; 125(4):272–6.
58. Mah J, Otsuka N, McLean J. An arthroscopic technique for the reduction and fixation of tibial-eminence fractures. J Pediatr Orthop 1996;16(1):119–21.
59. Hsu S. An easy and effective method for reattaching an anterior cruciate ligament avulsion fracture from the tibial eminence. Arthroscopy 2004;20(1):96–100.
60. Berg E. Comminuted tibial eminence anterior cruciate ligament avulsion fractures: failure of arthroscopic treatment. Arthroscopy 1993;9(4):446–50.
61. Park H, Urabe K, Naruse K, et al. Arthroscopic evaluation after surgical repair of intercondylar eminence fractures. Arch Orthop Trauma Surg 2007;127(9):753–7.
62. Matthews D, Geissler W. Arthroscopic suture fixation of displaced tibial eminence fractures. Arthroscopy 1994;10(4):418–23.
63. Ahn J, Lee YS, Lee DH, et al. Arthroscopic physeal sparing all inside repair of the tibial avulsion fracture in the anterior cruciate ligament: technical note. Arch Orthop Trauma Surg 2008;128(11):1309–12.
64. Hirschmann M, Mayer RR, Kentsch A, et al. Physeal sparing arthroscopic fixation of displaced tibial eminence fractures: a new surgical technique. Knee Surg Sports Traumatol Arthrosc 2009;17(7):741–7.
65. Huang T, Hsu KY, Cheng CY, et al. Arthroscopic suture fixation of tibial eminence avulsion fractures. Arthroscopy 2008;24(11):1232–8.
66. Lubowitz J, Grauer J. Arthroscopic treatment of anterior cruciate ligament avulsion. Clin Orthop Relat Res 1993;(294):242–6.
67. Doral M, Atay OA, Leblebicioglu G, et al. Arthroscopic fixation of the fractures of the intercondylar eminence via transquadricipital tendinous portal. Knee Surg Sports Traumatol Arthrosc 2001;9(6):346–9.

68. Reynders P, Reynders K, Broos P. Pediatric and adolescent tibial eminence fractures: arthroscopic cannulated screw fixation. L Trauma 2002;53(1):49–54.

69. Liljeros K. Arthroscopic fixation of anterior tibial spine fractures with bioabsorbable nails in skeletally immature patients. Am J Sports Med 2009;37(5):923–8.

70. Vega J, Irribarra LA, Baar AK, et al. Arthroscopic fixation of displaced tibial eminence fractures: a new growth plate-sparing method. Arthroscopy 2008;24(11):1239–43.

71. Lu XW, Hu XP, Jin C, et al. Reduction and fixation of the avulsion fracture of the tibial eminence using mini-open technique. Knee Surg Sports Traumatol Arthrosc 2010. [Epub ahead of print].

72. In Y, Kim JM, Woo YK, et al. Arthroscopic fixation of anterior cruciate ligament tibial avulsion fractures using bioabsorbable suture anchors. Knee Surg Sports Traumatol Arthrosc 2008;16(3):286–9.

73. Louis M, Guillaume JM, Launay F, et al. Surgical management of type II tibial intercondylar eminence fractures in children. J Pediatr Orthop B 2008;17(5):231–5.

74. Mahar A, Duncan D, Oka R, et al. Biomechanical comparison of four different fixation techniques for pediatric tibial eminence avulsion fractures. J Pediatr Orthop 2008; 28(2):159–62.

75. Eggers A, Becker C, Weimann A, et al. Biomechanical evaluation of different fixation methods for tibial eminence fractures. Am J Sports Med 2007;35(3):404–10.

76. Tsukada H, Ishibashi Y, Tsuda E, et al. A biomechanical comparison of repair techniques for anterior cruciate ligament tibial avulsion fracture under cyclic loading. Arthroscopy 2005;21(10):1197–201.

77. Bong M, Romero A, Kubiak E, et al. Suture versus screw fixation of displaced tibial eminence fractures: a biomechanical comparison. Arthroscopy 2005;21(10):1172–6.

78. Tsai T. Malpractice of epiphyseal cannulated screw fixation in a child with avulsion fracture of the tibial eminence complicating with lack of knee extension and distal femoral fracture. J Med Sci 2009;29(5):289–292.

79. Mylle J, Reynders P, Broos P. Transepiphysial fixation of anterior cruciate avulsion in a child. Report of a complication and review of the literature. Arch Orthop Trauma Surg 1993;112(2):101–3.

80. Anderson AF, Anderson CN. Anterior cruciate ligament injuries with bony avulsion. In: Lieberman JR, Berry DJ, Azar FM, editors. AAOS Advanced Reconstruction: Knee. Rosemont: AAOS; 2011. p. 603–12.

81. Vander Have K, Ganley TJ, Kocher MS, et al. Arthrofibrosis after surgical fixation of tibial eminence fractures in children and adolescents. Am J Sports Med 2010;38(2): 298–301.

82. Panni A, Milano G, Tartarone M, et al. Arthroscopic treatment of malunited and nonunited avulsion fractures of the anterior tibial spine. Arthroscopy 1998;14(3):233–40.

83. Luger EJ, Arbel R, Eichenblat MS, et al. Femoral notchplasty in the treatment of malunited intercondylar eminence fractures of the tibia. Arthroscopy 1994;10(5): 550–1.

Partial Tears of the Anterior Cruciate Ligament in Children and Adolescents

Michael T. Busch, MD[a], Meagan D. Fernandez, DO[b],*,
Chad Aarons, MD[c]

KEYWORDS
- ACL • Adolescent • Partial tear ACL
- Anteromedial bundle tear • Skeletally immature knee

Treatment of anterior cruciate ligament (ACL) tears in growing youths has evolved considerably over the past decade. There is a growing trend toward operative stabilization, because studies show the risks of not treating these injuries. We have gained experience on techniques that reduce the risk of surgical injury to the growing physis. Even for the complete tear of the ACL, controversies continue. Is there any role for nonoperative care? Is it safe to cross an open physis and before or after what age? How do we best determine skeletal maturity and remaining growth potential? Which "physeal-sparing" procedures best reproduce the native anatomy and therefore normal mechanics? Although the quantity and quality of scientifically sound information available to us limits our ability to be definitive, this article addresses the reliable scientific data that is available as well as expert experience and opinion.

Published data regarding partial ACL injury, particularly in youths, are limited and opinions differ regarding diagnosis and treatment. The partial ACL injury debate starts with the fundamentals of definition and diagnosis, which makes the process of providing the patient with informed conclusions and treatment algorithms challenging. Nevertheless, partial injuries are a reality and clinical decisions must be made based on the sound principles and the best available data.

No support or funds have been received for this work.
The authors have nothing to disclose.
[a] Children's Healthcare of Atlanta, 5445 Meridian Mark Road, Street 250, Atlanta, GA 30342, USA
[b] Department of Orthopaedic Surgery, Geisinger Medical Center, 100 North Academy Avenue, MC2130, Danville, PA 17822, USA
[c] Tuckahoe Orthopaedic Associates, 1501 Maple Avenue, Suite 200, Richmond, VA 23226, USA
* Corresponding author.
E-mail address: mdelbaggio@aol.com

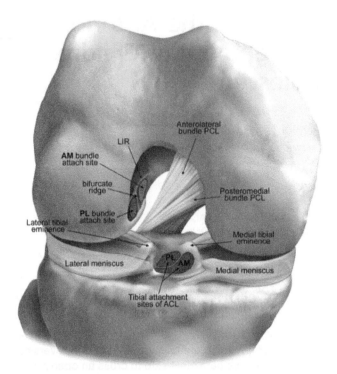

Fig. 1. Anatomic view of a right knee demonstrating pertinent arthroscopic landmarks on the femur and tibia, the tibial and femoral ACL bundle attachments, and the relationship of the tibial and femoral ACL attachments to each other in the native knee. AM, anteromedial bundle; LIR, lateral intercondylar ridge; PCL, posterior cruciate ligament; PL, posterolateral bundle. (*From* Ziegler CG, Petrini SD, Westerhasu BD, et al. Arthroscopically pertinent landmarks for tunnel positioning in single-bundle and double-bundle anterior cruciate ligament reconstructions. Am J Sports Med 2011;39:743–52.)

DEFINITION

In 1936, Weber first described 2 functional bundles of the ACL.[1] It has been well-recognized since then that the ACL consists of the anteromedial and postero-lateral bundles, so named for the orientation of their tibial insertions (**Fig. 1**).

Selective injury to 1 of the bundles of the ACL seems to be related to the position of the knee when the injury occurs.[2–4] The anteromedial bundle tightens in flexion, whereas the posterolateral bundle relaxes. The posterolateral bundle tightens in extension and internal rotation.

Rupture of the anteromedial bundle allows an increase in anterior translation when the knee is in flexion. There is little or no increased laxity in hyperextension, and little or no clinically significant rotational instability.[5] Hyperextension and internal rotation place the posterolateral bundle under tension and therefore at greater risk for injury. Rupture of the posterolateral bundle may result in an increase in hyperextension, an increase in anterior translation with the knee in extension, an increase in external and internal rotation with the knee in extension, and an increase in external rotation with the knee in 45° of flexion.[5]

Although Darach first described partial ACL tears more than 75 years ago, the literature remains limited and inconsistent for partial ACL tears. In all age groups, the reported incidence of partial ACL tears ranges from 10% to 50%; some physicians question the value of even making this distinction because clinicians disagree on the definition, diagnostic criteria, natural history, and the effective treatment options.

So, the controversies begin with the very definition of a partial tear of the ACL. That definition varies from bleeding at the femoral attachment of the ACL to total rupture of either the anteromedial or posterolateral bundles. What percentage of torn fibers constitutes a partial tear of the ACL? Opinions have ranged from tears of 25% to 75%.[6–8]

DIAGNOSIS

How do we assess the extent of injury? Methods include physical examination, devices designed to quantify anterior translation, advanced imaging, and intraoperative arthroscopic findings. The Lachman pivot shift and anterior drawer tests have been studied for their ability to identify complete tears of the ACL. Katz and colleagues[9] compared these 3 examinations in acute and chronic knee injuries.[9] All examinations were performed under anesthesia and confirmed on arthroscopy. When including all ACL injuries, regardless of chronicity, the Lachman test was 82% sensitive and 97% specific. The anterior drawer sign was 41% sensitive and 93% specific. The pivot shift was 82% sensitive and 98% specific. These data have to be cautiously applied to clinical practice because this study was done with patients under general anesthesia and were based on the ability to diagnose a complete tear of the ACL. Donaldson and colleagues[10] performed a retrospective study on 100 patients with arthroscopically documented ACL tears. Both the preoperative examination and examination under anesthesia were reviewed to assess accuracy. The preoperative examination (without anesthesia) found that 98% of the Lachman tests, 54% of the anterior drawer tests, and 27% of the pivot shifts were positive. Under anesthesia, 100% of the Lachman tests, 81% of anterior drawer tests, and 100% of pivot shift tests were positive.[11]

On a standard physical examination, both Lachman and pivot shift testing often fail to identify a partial tear of the ACL, even when up to 75% of the ligament is torn.[12] Sandberg and Balkfors[8] showed that stability tests in partial tears of the ACL could be initially negative and transition to positive during their follow-up period of 18 months. Crain and colleagues showed that any intact fibers to the roof of the intercondylar notch, whether scar or native tissue, provided significant support. They found that repeat sectioning of these fibers resulted in a significant increase in anterior translation of the knee. In an incomplete injury, the remaining ACL fibers may produce a false-negative examination, rendering the physical examination less effective in diagnosing partial ACL tears.[7]

Devices have been developed to provide more sensitive and objective measurement than the physical findings. Such quantitative assessment of anterior tibial translation can be imprecise, subjective, and poorly reproducible.[11,13] The KT-1000 arthrometer, introduced in the early 1980s by Daniel and colleagues,[14] is the most widely used knee ligament testing system, largely because of its ease of use. It remains a common reference instrument for many scientific papers.[14] However, the KT-1000 is operator dependent and imprecise standardization of limb alignment and hamstring contraction during measurement can affect reproducibility.

Robert and colleagues[15] recently introduced the GeNouRoB device with hopes of decreasing false-negative results.[15] This device standardizes the position of the knee during testing. By assessing muscular activity in the hamstrings, the GeNouRoB attempts to eliminate their resistance to anterior tibial translation. Initial studies have shown 80% sensitivity and 87% specificity for the diagnosis of an isolated antero-medial bundle tear. However, the availability of having such a quantitative measuring device in every office seems to be both cost and time prohibitive.

Imaging experts have studied a number of findings in an attempt to identify incomplete injuries of the ACL. Magnetic resonance imaging (MRI) can attempt to quantitate the percentage of intact fibers after an injury. Oblique coronal MRI imaging seems to be the most accurate.[16,17] Chen and colleagues[18] described direct and indirect signs associated with a partial ACL tear. Residual straight and tight ACL fibers, in at least 1 pulse sequence, was frequently detected in partial ACL tears. Findings that are common in complete ACL tears include the empty notch sign, a wavy contour of ACL, bone contusion of the lateral compartment, and posterior horn tears of the lateral meniscus. Compared with chronic partial ACL tears, chronic complete tears have a more acute posterior cruciate ligament angle.

Direct arthroscopic visualization is a more definitive method of evaluation, but certain types of partial ACL tears pose challenges when assessing for intact fibers even using this method. Sonnery-Cottet and colleagues[19] showed that identifying an isolated posterolateral bundle tear is more difficult than identifying an anteromedial bundle tear on standard arthroscopy. More accurate assessment of the posterolateral bundle may be obtained with the patient's leg in Cabot's position (figure 4 position).

Crain and colleagues[20] also graded ACL tears arthroscopically. They examined variations in the ACL tear pattern and their relationships with anterior laxity. They found 4 distinct groups: ACL remnant scarring to the PCL (38%), ACL remnant scarring to the roof of the notch (8%), ACL remnant scarring to the lateral femoral condyle (12%), and no identifiable ligament tissue remaining (42%). Based on their criteria, 58% of all ACL tears were labeled partial tears, but at what point does a "partially torn" ACL become clinically ineffective and therefore virtually a complete tear?

DeFranco and Bach[21] combined several of the aforementioned criteria to create a more functional definition of partial ACL tears.[21] They defined a partial tear as existing if the following 4 criteria are met: (1) An asymmetric Lachman-test is present (as compared with the unaffected knee), (2) a negative pivot shift with the patient under anesthesia, (3) a low-grade KT-1000 measurement (≤3 mm), and (4) arthroscopic evidence of an incomplete ACL injury. In their opinion, the absence of a pivot shift indicates a stable or functional partial tear of the ACL, whereas the presence of pivot shifting signifies a nonfunctional or unstable ligament. Even if the remaining ACL fibers adequately stabilize the knee for the pivot shift examination, and for daily activities, one may question the amount of load those partially injured bundles will tolerate during demanding activities such as sports.

PROGNOSIS

Once a partial tear of the ACL is identified, how should it be treated? To accurately assess whether a treatment for a partial ACL tear is effective, we must know the natural history of the injury. Once again, our ability to be definitive is limited by the reliable information available to us. There are relatively few true natural history studies; most so titled include a hodgepodge of nonoperatively treated patients. Natural history studies, with reasonable numbers of subjects, commonly mix adults and children, and few include patients younger than 13. Bone ages are rarely documented for these studies, so the number of skeletally immature patients is uncertain. In general, children have better healing potential than adults; however, we do not know for certain whether prepubescent, pubescent, and fully mature youths differ in their ability to heal or compensate for partial ACL injuries.

Some studies report good to excellent functional results in adults with mild laxity, even if they maintain or slightly reduce their activity level.[7,8,22–25] Others have suggested that many partial tears function like complete injuries, and therefore have a poor prognosis.[25,26]

The degree of laxity can increase after the diagnosis of a partial ACL tear, and it is often presumed that the partial tear progressed to complete tear. This has been reported in 14% to 56% of injuries followed for 1.5 to 5.3 years after nonoperative management.[25,27–30] One explanation of the progression to complete tear is that the vascular supply of the remaining ligament was compromised at the time of injury. It is hypothesized that ischemic necrosis weakens the remaining ligament over time.[6,26] Perhaps the weakened ligament is simply not robust enough to withstand the loads applied during activities, so it fails because of additional minor injuries or from chronic stresses.

TREATMENT

Kocher and colleagues[31] studied 45 skeletally mature and immature patients ($<$18 years old) diagnosed to have a partial ACL injury. Their criteria for diagnosis was an injury that resulted in hemarthrosis, pertinent MRI signal changes, normal to minimally positive Lachman and pivot shift examinations, and an arthroscopically documented partial ACL tear. All patients were initially treated with a structured rehabilitation program. They were all followed for a minimum of 2 years. Fourteen patients (31%) underwent subsequent ACL reconstruction. The risk factors for needing eventual reconstruction included tears that involved more than 50% of the cross-sectional area, tears that predominantly involved the posterolateral bundle, a mildly positive pivot shift test, and older chronologic and skeletal ages. They concluded that nonoperative management of partial ACL tears in children and adolescents, 14 years of skeletal age or younger, with normal or near-normal Lachman and pivot shift results could be successful. They recommended reconstruction for older adolescent athletes (15- to 17-year-olds), those with greater than 50% of the ligament injured, and for those with tears that were predominantly of the posterolateral bundle. To date, this is the only study of partial ACL tears in an exclusively pediatric cohort.

Reconstruction of the partially injured ACL includes the option of replacing 1 bundle while sparing the less injured bundle. Those who prefer sparing the intact bundle point out that the remaining ACL fibers have mechanoreceptors that are normally involved in providing proprioception for the knee.[32–34] One study even suggested that neural elements from the intact fibers may repopulate the graft.[35] It has also been suggested that the blood supply of the spared bundle may help with healing of the graft.[36] Regardless of whether these benefits occur, single bundle replacement seems to be a viable option. Sonnery-Cottet and colleagues[37] published their results of single bundle replacement in 36 patients. They reported a decrease of anterior translation from 4.8 to 0.8 mm after anteromedial bundle reconstruction.

There are, however, down sides to selective bundle reconstruction. Abundant amounts of tissue in the intercondylar notch can limit knee motion. A relatively smaller graft might ameliorate impingement, but reduces graft strength. Proponents of complete ligament reconstruction also point out that the force needed to rupture an ACL bundle probably results in substantial interstitial damage in the remaining bundle. Ligament fibers may elongate by more than 50% compared with their resting length prior to ultimate failure.[6] So, significant microscopic damage may be present, yet not readily apparent to visual inspection of the ligament. Many contend that a full substitution graft better serves the patient than sparing a macroscopically intact but presumably damaged bundle.

SUMMARY

The treatment of partial ACL tears in the adult population remains somewhat controversial; the treatment in children is even more uncertain because there is a paucity of high-quality information on the subject. There are no uniform criteria for the diagnosis of a partial injury to the ACL and there is no certain method for assessing the biological and mechanical extent of injury when a portion of the ACL remains intact. There seems to be a subset of patients with partial ACL injuries who do well without a operative reconstruction. The challenge is to reliably identify those individuals and to devise effective treatment recommendations for them. Characteristics of those who have a more favorable prognosis when treated without reconstruction include younger age, lower demand activities, a mildly positive Lachman with a negative pivot shift, and less than 50% disruption by MRI and/or arthroscopy. In partial ACL injuries, surgical reconstruction involving preservation of the less injured bundle is an option; however, a single bundle reconstruction is potentially weaker and clinically unproven. Established principles apply to active otherwise healthy young patients and dictate that functional instability should be treated by reconstruction since the natural history of functionally unstable young patients with ACL compromise is unfavorable and can result in potentially irreversible meniscus and articular cartilage injury.

REFERENCES

1. Bercovy M, Weber E. [Evaluation of laxity, rigidity and compliance of the normal and pathological knee. Application to survival curves of ligamentoplasties]. Rev Chir Orthop Reparatrice Appar Mot 1995;81(2):114–27 [in French].
2. Livesay GA, Fujie H, Kashiwaguchi S, et al. Determination of the in situ forces and force distribution within the human anterior cruciate ligament. Ann Biomed Eng 1995;23(4):467–74.
3. Rudy TW, Livesay GA, Woo SL, et al. A combined robotic/universal force sensor approach to determine in situ forces of knee ligaments. J Biomech 1996;29(10): 1357–60.
4. Boisgard S, Levai JP, Geiger B, et al. Study of the variations in length of the anterior cruciate ligament during flexion of the knee: use of a 3D model reconstructed from MRI sections. Surg Radiol Anat 1999;21(5):313–7.
5. Furman W, Marshall JL, Girgis FG. The anterior cruciate ligament. A functional analysis based on postmortem studies. J Bone Joint Surg Am 1976;58(2):179–85.
6. Noyes FR, Mooar LA, Moorman CT 3rd, et al. Partial tears of the anterior cruciate ligament. Progression to complete ligament deficiency. J Bone Joint Surg Br 1989; 71(5):825–33.
7. Odensten M, Lysholm J, Gillquist J. The course of partial anterior cruciate ligament ruptures. Am J Sports Med 1985;13(3):183–6.
8. Sandberg R, Balkfors B. Partial rupture of the anterior cruciate ligament. Natural course. Clin Orthop Relat Res 1987(220):176–8.
9. Katz JW, Fingeroth RJ. The diagnostic accuracy of ruptures of the anterior cruciate ligament comparing the Lachman test, the anterior drawer sign, and the pivot shift test in acute and chronic knee injuries. Am J Sports Med 1986;14(1):88–91.
10. Donaldson WF 3rd, Warren RF, Wickiewicz T. A comparison of acute anterior cruciate ligament examinations. Initial versus examination under anesthesia. Am J Sports Med 1985;13(1):5–10.

11. Benvenuti JF, Vallotton JA, Meystre JL, et al. Objective assessment of the anterior tibial translation in Lachman test position. Comparison between three types of measurement. Knee Surg Sports Traumatol Arthrosc 1998;6(4):215–9.
12. Hole RL, Lintner DM, Kamaric E, et al. Increased tibial translation after partial sectioning of the anterior cruciate ligament. The posterolateral bundle. Am J Sports Med 1996;24(4):556–60.
13. Wiertsema SH, van Hooff HJ, Migchelsen LA, et al. Reliability of the KT1000 arthrometer and the Lachman test in patients with an ACL rupture. Knee 2008;15(2):107–10.
14. Daniel DM, Stone ML, Sachs R, et al. Instrumented measurement of anterior knee laxity in patients with acute anterior cruciate ligament disruption. Am J Sports Med 1985;13(6):401–7.
15. Robert H, Nouveau S, Gageot S, et al. A new knee arthrometer, the GNRB: experience in ACL complete and partial tears. Orthop Traumatol Surg Res 2009;95(3): 171–6.
16. Noyes FR, Mooar PA, Matthews DS, et al. The symptomatic anterior cruciate-deficient knee. Part I: the long-term functional disability in athletically active individuals. J Bone Joint Surg Am 1983;65(2):154–62.
17. Hong SH, Choi JY, Lee GK, et al. Grading of anterior cruciate ligament injury. Diagnostic efficacy of oblique coronal magnetic resonance imaging of the knee. J Comput Assist Tomogr 2003;27(5):814–9.
18. Chen WT, Shih TT, Tu HY, et al. Partial and complete tear of the anterior cruciate ligament. Acta Radiol 2002;43(5):511–6.
19. Sonnery-Cottet B, Barth J, Graveleau N, et al. Arthroscopic identification of isolated tear of the posterolateral bundle of the anterior cruciate ligament. Arthroscopy 2009;25(7):728–32.
20. Crain EH, Fithian DC, Paxton EW, et al. Variation in anterior cruciate ligament scar pattern: does the scar pattern affect anterior laxity in anterior cruciate ligament-deficient knees? Arthroscopy 2005;21(1):19–24.
21. DeFranco MJ, Bach BR, Jr. A comprehensive review of partial anterior cruciate ligament tears. J Bone Joint Surg Am 2009;91(1):198–208.
22. Kannus P, Jarvinen M. Conservatively treated tears of the anterior cruciate ligament. Long-term results. J Bone Joint Surg Am 1987;69(7):1007–12.
23. Neusel E, Maibaum S, Rompe G. Five-year results of conservatively treated tears of the anterior cruciate ligament. Arch Orthop Trauma Surg 1996;115(6):332–6.
24. Sommerlath K, Odensten M, Lysholm J. The late course of acute partial anterior cruciate ligament tears. A nine to 15-year follow-up evaluation. Clin Orthop Relat Res 1992(281):152–8.
25. Bak K, Scavenius M, Hansen S, et al. Isolated partial rupture of the anterior cruciate ligament. Long-term follow-up of 56 cases. Knee Surg Sports Traumatol Arthrosc 1997;5(2):66–71.
26. Lintner DM, Kamaric E, Moseley JB, et al. Partial tears of the anterior cruciate ligament. Are they clinically detectable? Am J Sports Med 1995;23(1):111–8.
27. Fritschy D, Panoussopoulos A, Wallensten R, et al. Can we predict the outcome of a partial rupture of the anterior cruciate ligament? A prospective study of 43 cases. Knee Surg Sports Traumatol Arthrosc 1997;5(1):2–5.
28. Lehnert M, Eisenschenk A, Zellner A. Results of conservative treatment of partial tears of the anterior cruciate ligament. Int Orthop 1993;17(4):219–23.
29. Barrack RL, Buckley SL, Bruckner JD, et al. Partial versus complete acute anterior cruciate ligament tears. The results of nonoperative treatment. J Bone Joint Surg Br 1990;72(4):622–4.

30. Fruensgaard S, Johannsen HV. Incomplete ruptures of the anterior cruciate ligament. J Bone Joint Surg Br 1989;71(3):526–30.
31. Kocher MS, Micheli LJ, Zurakowski D, et al. Partial tears of the anterior cruciate ligament in children and adolescents. Am J Sports Med 2002;30(5):697–703.
32. Schultz RA, Miller DC, Kerr CS, et al. Mechanoreceptors in human cruciate ligaments. A histological study. J Bone Joint Surg Am 1984;66(7):1072–6.
33. Schutte MJ, Dabezies EJ, Zimny ML, et al. Neural anatomy of the human anterior cruciate ligament. J Bone Joint Surg Am 1987;69(2):243–7.
34. Denti M, Monteleone M, Berardi A, et al. Anterior cruciate ligament mechanoreceptors. Histologic studies on lesions and reconstruction. Clin Orthop Relat Res 1994(308):29–32.
35. Georgoulis AD, Pappa L, Moebius U, et al. The presence of proprioceptive mechanoreceptors in the remnants of the ruptured ACL as a possible source of re-innervation of the ACL autograft. Knee Surg Sports Traumatol Arthrosc 2001;9(6):364–8.
36. Deie M, Ochi M, Ikuta Y. High intrinsic healing potential of human anterior cruciate ligament. Organ culture experiments. Acta Orthop Scand 1995;66(1):28–32.
37. Sonnery-Cottet B, Lavoie F, Ogassawara R, et al. Selective anteromedial bundle reconstruction in partial ACL tears: a series of 36 patients with mean 24 months follow-up. Knee Surg Sports Traumatol Arthrosc 2010;18(1):47–51.

Reconstruction of Anterior Cruciate Ligament in Children: Hamstring versus Bone Patella Tendon Bone Graft

James H.P. Hui, MBBS, FRCS, MD[a],*,
Ashwin Chowdhary, MBBS, D Orth, MS Orth, MRCS[b]

KEYWORDS
- Anterior cruciate ligament • Children • Hamstring
- BTB graft

Tears of the anterior cruciate ligament (ACL) are uncommon[1,2] injuries in the skeletally immature population. They were once thought to occur only after closure of the growth plate.[3] However, recent studies have reported mid-substance tears of the ACL with increasing frequency[4,5] in children. This may be due to increased awareness, improved imaging techniques,[6] and increased participation in sports at an earlier age.

Nonoperative treatment of such injuries has shown poor results in the long term, with problems of poor long-term function,[7] instability,[5,8] meniscus tears,[9] osteochondral fractures,[7] osteoarthritic changes,[7,8] and inability to return to pre-injury level of sports.[9] This may be reserved as a temporary procedure to avoid risks of possible growth disturbances or in partial ruptures of ACL without instability.[10] Direct primary repair[11] and extra-articular procedures have not been very successful in providing stability after mid-substance tears of ACL.

The goal of ACL reconstruction is restoration of functional knee stability by replacing the injured ligament with graft material. Commonly used graft materials include the hamstrings and the bone patella tendon autografts. Rarely, Achilles tendon may be used. Allografts, synthetic grafts, and ligament augmentation devices are not commonly used for the pediatric population.

No support or funds have been received for this work.
The authors have nothing to disclose.
[a] Division of Paediatric Orthopaedics, National University Hospital, University Orthopaedics and HRM Cluster, 5, Lower Kent Ridge Road, Kent Ridge Wing 2, Level 3, 119074, Singapore
[b] Division of Paediatric Orthopaedics, National University Hospital, University Orthopaedics and HRM Cluster, 5, Lower Kent Ridge Road, Kent Ridge Wing 2, Level 3, 119074, Singapore
* Corresponding author.
E-mail address: James_hui@nuhs.edu.sg

In skeletally mature adolescents, standard arthroscopically assisted techniques using hamstrings or bone-patellar tendon-bone (BTB) grafts can be used to reconstruct the ACL. In the skeletally immature, various techniques such as physeal sparing and partial transphyseal techniques have been described to limit the potential of physeal injury. Complete transphyseal reconstructions have the potential of causing physeal damage.[12,13] However, recent studies[7,14,15] have suggested that these might be safe. Growth disturbances are likely to occur if the damage to the physis is more than 9% of its cross-sectional area.[13,16] Janarv and colleagues[16] have shown that the transphyseal tunnels in ACL reconstructions occupy only 3% to 4% of the cross-sectional area of the physes. According to Beasley and Chudik,[17] small tunnels that are centrally placed and filled with soft tissue are less likely to cause growth disturbances unlike eccentrically placed tunnels or those filled with cancellous bone. Soft tissue across an open physis usually prevents its closure as shown classically by Langenskiold[18] for treatment of physeal bars. Hamstrings serve well as a soft tissue graft and allow their placement across the physes. In a study of transphyseal ACL reconstruction in canine models, Edwards and colleagues[12] have shown that significant growth disturbances occurred only when tendons were placed across the physes in excessive tension. Kocher and colleagues[19] have reported that growth disturbances may be associated with bone plugs (of BTB graft) or fixation hardware across the physis.

GRAFT HEALING/STRENGTH AND STIFFNESS

The strength of the graft fixation complex must be considered when choosing between the type of graft, be it the hamstrings or the BTB. The main factor affecting the structural strength of this complex in the initial weeks is not the strength of the graft but the fixation points, especially so on the tibial[20] side. Pinczewski and colleagues[21] found that after bone-to-bone or tendon-to-bone healing has taken place, usually at 6 to 15 weeks postoperatively, the fixation points are not the weakest link. In a study of graft-to-bone healing for ACL reconstructions in a canine model, Rodeo and colleagues[22] have shown that failure occurred by pull out of the tendon from bone tunnels in the first 8 weeks, whereas after 12 weeks, grafts usually failed because of mid-substance rupture of the grafts itself.

Bone-to-bone healing of BTB grafts has been shown to be faster than the healing of hamstrings grafts.[23] In animal models, Rodeo and colleagues[22] found that bone healing with a BTB graft usually occurred by 6 weeks, whereas tendon graft took up to approximately 12 weeks to heal. In a comparative study of intra-osseous healing of tendon grafts and BTB grafts for ACL reconstruction in dogs, Tomita and colleagues[24] have shown that tendon graft anchored to bone at 12 weeks, whereas BTB graft was anchored to bone as early as 3 weeks. They found the pull-out strength of BTB grafts to be superior to tendon grafts at 3 weeks after ACL reconstruction. They have also shown that healing of tendon grafts occurs by newly formed collagen fibers, whereas healing of BTB grafts occurs by new bone formation.

All grafted tendon tissue loses some of its initial strength during the healing period. In a study of ACL reconstruction in dogs, Butler[25] has shown that significant loss in structural mechanical and material properties of grafts occurred early after implantation. In another study, McFarland and colleagues[26] have shown grafts to become weaker by 4 weeks after implantation. According to Prodromos and Joyce,[27] they may retain only about half their initial strength in long-term follow-up. Therefore, an initial graft needs to be significantly stronger than the native ACL in order to produce an ultimate strength at least as strong as the original ACL. Noyes and colleagues[28] have shown that a 14- to 15-mm-wide BTB graft has a mean initial strength of 159%

to 168% of that of ACLs, whereas semitendinosus and gracilis tendons have a 70% and 49%, respectively, of the initial strength of ACLs. Thus after losing half of its strength, a BTB graft's final strength may be less than the original ACL strength, whereas a double or quadrupled hamstring graft will be stronger. In a biomechanical analysis of grafts harvested from cadaveric knees, Wilson and colleagues[29] have shown double-looped hamstring grafts to be significantly stronger than BTB grafts.

It is also important to consider the stiffness of the graft in addition to its strength. According to Dopirak and colleagues,[30] a graft that lacks stiffness may have a propensity to elongate, which could be manifest clinically as increased laxity. In a study on cadaveric knees, Rowden and colleagues[31] have shown the stiffness of ACL to be 306 ± 80 N/mm; Woo and colleagues[32] have found the same to be 242 ± 28 N/mm. In a study of BTB grafts from cadaveric knees, Cooper and colleagues[33] have shown the stiffness of a 10-mm patellar tendon graft to be around 455 N/mm. To and colleagues[34] have shown the stiffness of a double-looped hamstring graft to average at 954 ± 292 N/mm. Hence both the hamstring and the BTB grafts possess stiffness that exceeds that of the normal ACL, the 4-stranded hamstring graft being stiffer. Hamner and colleagues[35] also have shown 4-stranded hamstring grafts to be stiffer than BTB grafts. On the contrary, in a randomized prospective study, Beynnon and colleagues[36] showed that 2-stranded hamstring grafts produce more knee laxity than BTB grafts when measured with KT 1000 (MEDmetric(r) Corporation, San Diego, CA, USA) laxity meter and pivot shift grades. Pinczewski and colleagues[37] have also demonstrated that hamstring grafts resulted in increased laxity when compared with BTB grafts in the intermediate follow-up, although long-term results were similar. Others, such as Harilainen and colleagues,[38] Tow and colleagues,[39] Laxdal and coworkers,[40] Ejerhed and colleagues,[41] Jansson and colleagues,[42] and Sajovic and coworkers,[43] have not found statistically significant differences with respect to clinical and instrumented laxity testing between the hamstring and BTB grafts.

GRAFT MORPHOLOGICAL/HISTOLOGICAL CHARACTERISTICS AND LIGAMENTIZATION

Hamstrings and BTB grafts differ in their morphological and histological characteristics. Hadjicostas and colleagues[44] have done a comparative analysis of the thickness of collagen fibrils, fibril:interstitium ratio, density of blood vessels, density of fibroblasts, and distribution of the collagen fibrils in hamstring and patella tendons harvested from cadaveric knees. They have shown that the semitendinosus and gracilis tendons provide 20% and 30% more fibril:interstitium ratio compared with the patella tendon. Also, the density of fibroblasts in the semitendinosus and gracilis tendons was 50% and 35% more than the patella tendon, respectively. The thickness of the collagen fibrils, density of blood vessels, and distribution of the fibrils were similar in both the tendons. The hamstrings therefore, theoretically, have a potential advantage over the patella tendon graft of better remodeling and regeneration of the tissue.

The normal ACL has been shown to carry loads throughout the entire range of flexion and extension of the knee. This is accomplished by the recruitment of different fibers within the gross structure of the ACL as the knee joint moves. Operative reconstruction of ACL should aim at restoring the ability of the healed structure to recruit fibers throughout the full range of motion of the knee. According to Frank and Jackson,[23] hamstring graft, when compared with the BTB graft, has a theoretical advantage of recreating a multibundled structure that may be better suited for this purpose.

Ligamentization is the process by which a graft transforms into a structure that is similar histologically to the normal ACL. This has been conclusively shown to occur after ACL reconstruction with BTB graft. Using rabbit models, Amiel and colleagues[45] have shown the cell morphology of patella tendon to become ligamentous by 30 weeks as evidenced by the increased concentration of type 3 collagen, and a pattern of high dihydroxylysinonorleucine and low histidinohydroxymerodesmosine, which is seen in normal ACL. In canine models, Arnoczky and colleagues[46] have shown that the patella tendon grafts were completely ensheathed in a vascular synovial envelope by 6 weeks, and by 1 year their vascular and histological appearance resembled that of a normal ACL. Rougraff and colleagues[47] have described 4 stages in the ligamentization of human autogenous patellar tendon grafts, with the grafts becoming viable as early as 3 weeks postoperatively and the whole process of ligamentization taking up to 3 years to complete. Recent data demonstrate that ligamentization occurs after ACL reconstruction with hamstring tendon grafts as well. Using sheep models for ACL reconstructions, Goradia and colleagues[48] have shown that hamstring autografts transform into a structure that is histologically similar to the normal ACL by 1 year, as has been described for patellar tendon grafts. Lane and colleagues[49] have evaluated the histological and biochemical changes that occurred in a hamstring autograft in a human patient and have found the appearance and biochemical properties of the hamstring autograft and the native ACL to be similar.

POTENTIAL COMPLICATIONS

Complications may occur both with the BTB or hamstrings. In a study of 604 patients who underwent ACL reconstruction using BTB grafts, Kartus and colleagues[50] have described various complications including extension deficit of more than 5 degrees, anterior knee pain, anterior knee insensitivity, and problems with knee walking. Järvela and colleagues[51] evaluated 91 patients who had ACL reconstruction with BTB grafts and found anterior knee pain as a cause of patient dissatisfaction. Shelbourne and Trumper[52] followed up 602 patients who had ACL reconstruction with BTB grafts and suggested obtaining full knee hyperextension postoperatively to decrease the incidence of anterior knee pain. However, in a randomized prospective study on 164 patients, Eriksson and colleagues[53] did not find any significant difference in anterior knee pain with the use of BTB grafts when compared with hamstring grafts. They have reported loss of terminal extension with the use of BTB grafts. In a randomized prospective trial of 71 patients, Ejerhed and colleagues[41] found donor site morbidity and poorer knee-walking ability to be associated with BTB grafts. Laxdal and colleagues[40] have described similar problems of increased discomfort during knee walking with the uses of BTB grafts. Corry and colleagues,[54] Otto and colleagues,[55] and Sachs and colleagues[56] have shown increased incidences of quadriceps wasting and donor site morbidity with the use of BTB grafts. Bonamo and colleagues[57] and Langan and Fontanetta[58] have reported rupture of the donor patella tendon after BTB harvesting. Piva and colleagues,[59] Brownstein and Bronner,[60] and Viola and Vianello[61] have found fractures of patella to be associated with BTB grafts. Voos and colleagues[62] have reported a complex intraarticular proximal tibia fracture in a patient who had ACL reconstruction with autologous BTB graft. According to Kocher and colleagues,[19] genu recurvatum may occur if the tibial apophysis is injured during BTB graft harvesting. Viola and colleagues[63] and Segawa and colleagues[64] report weakness of tibial internal rotation after harvesting of hamstring grafts. Gobbi[65] has shown that loss of deep knee flexion and decreased knee flexion strength may be associated with hamstring grafts.

REFERENCES

1. De Lee JC, Curtis R. Anterior cruciate insufficiency in children. Clin Orthop 1983;172: 122–9.
2. Lipscomb AB, Anderson AF. Tears of the anterior cruciate ligament in adolescents. J Bone Joint Surg Am 1986;68:19–28.
3. Rang M, editor. Children's fractures. Philadelphia: JB Lippincott; 1983. p. 290.
4. Dorizas JA, Stanitski CL. Anterior cruciate ligament injury in the skeletally immature. Orthop Clin North Am 2003;34(3):355–63.
5. McCarroll JR, Rettig AC, Shelbourne KD. Anterior cruciate ligament injuries in the young adult with open physes. Am J Sports Med 1988;16:44–7.
6. Stanitski CL. Anterior cruciate ligament injury in the skeletally immature patient: diagnosis and treatment. J Am Acad Orthop Surg 1995;3:146–58.
7. Aichroth PM, Patel DV, Zorilla P. The natural history and treatment of rupture of the anterior cruciate ligament in children and adolescents. J Bone Joint Surg Br 2002;84-B:38–41.
8. Kannus P, Jarvinen M. Knee ligament injuries in adolescents: eight year follow-up of conservative treatment. J Bone Joint Surg Br 1988;70:772–6.
9. Mizuta H, Kubota K, Shiraishi M, et al. The conservative treatment of complete tears of anterior cruciate ligament in skeletally immature patients. J Bone Joint Surg Br 1995;77:890–4.
10. Kocher MS, Micheli LJ, Zurakowski D, et al. Partial tears of the anterior cruciate ligament in children and adolescents. Am J Sports Med 2002;30(5):697–703.
11. Engebretsen L, Svenningsen S, Benum P. Poor results of anterior cruciate ligament repair in adolescence. Acta Ortop Scand 1988;59:684–6.
12. Edwards TB, Greene CC, Baratta RV, et al. The effect of placing a tensioned graft across open growth plates. A gross and histologic analysis. J Bone Joint Surg Am 2001;83:725–34.
13. Guzzanti V, Falciglia F, Gigante A, et al. The effect of intra-articular ACL reconstruction on the growth plates of rabbits. J Bone Joint Surg 1994;76-B:960–3.
14. Aronowitz ER, Ganley TJ, Goode JR, et al. Anterior cruciate ligament reconstruction in adolescents with open physes. Am J Sports Med 2000;28(2):168–75.
15. Aichroth PM, Patel DV, Zorrilla P. The natural history and treatment of rupture of the anterior cruciate ligament in children and adolescents. A prospective review. J Bone Joint Surg Br 2002;84(1):38–41.
16. Janarv PM, Nystrom A, Werner S, et al. Anterior cruciate ligament injuries in skeletally immature patients. J Pediatr Orthop 1996;16:673–7.
17. Beasley LS, Chudik SC. Anterior cruciate ligament injury in children: update of current treatment options. Curr Opin Pediatr 2003;15:45–52.
18. Langenskiold A. An operation for partial closure of an epiphyseal plate in children and its experimental basis. J Bone Joint Surg 1975;57(B):325–30.
19. Kocher MS, Saxon HS, Hovis WD, et al. Management and complications of anterior cruciate ligament injuries in skeletally immature patients: survey of the Herodicus Society and the ACL Study Group. J Pediatr Orthop 2002;22(4):452–7.
20. Scheffler SU, Südkamp NP, Göckenjan A, et al. Biomechanical comparison of hamstring and patellar tendon graft anterior cruciate ligament reconstruction techniques: the impact of fixation level and fixation method under cyclic loading. Arthroscopy 2002;18(3):304–15.
21. Pinczewski LA, Clingeleffer AJ, Otto DD, et al. Integration of hamstring tendon graft with bone in reconstruction of the anterior cruciate ligament. Arthroscopy 1997;13: 641–3.

22. Rodeo SA, Arnoczky SP, Torzilli PA, et al. Tendon-healing in a bone tunnel. A biomechanical and histological study in the dog. J Bone Joint Surg Am 1993;75: 1795–803.

23. Frank CB, Jackson DW. The science of reconstruction of the anterior cruciate ligament. J Bone Joint Surg Am 1997;79(10):1556–76.

24. Tomita F, Yasuda K, Mikami S, et al. Comparisons of intraosseous graft healing between the doubled flexor tendon graft and the bone-patellar tendon-bone graft in anterior cruciate ligament reconstruction. Arthroscopy 2001;17(5):461–76.

25. Butler DL. Anterior cruciate ligament: its normal response and replacement. J Orthop Res 1989;7(6):910–21.

26. McFarland EG, Morrey BF, An KN, et al. The relationship of vascularity and water content to tensile strength in a patellar tendon replacement of the anterior cruciate in dogs. Am J Sports Med 1986;14(6):436–48.

27. Prodromos CC, Joyce BT. The relative strengths of anterior cruciate ligament autografts and allografts. In: Prodromos CC, editor. The anterior cruciate ligament: reconstruction and basic science. Philadelphia (PA): Elsevier; 2008. p. 84–7. Chapter 10.

28. Noyes FR, Butler DL, Grood ES, et al. Biomechanical analysis of human ligament grafts used in knee-ligament repairs and reconstructions. J Bone Joint Surg Am 1984;66:344–52.

29. Wilson TW, Zafuta MP, Zobitz M. A biomechanical analysis of matched bone-patellar tendon-bone and double-looped semitendinosus and gracilis tendon grafts. J Sports Med 1999;27(2):202–7.

30. Dopirak RM, Adamany DC, Steensen RN. A comparison of autogenous patellar tendon and hamstring tendon grafts for anterior cruciate ligament reconstruction. Orthopedics 2004;27(8):837–42 [quiz: 843–4].

31. Rowden NJ, Sher D, Rogers GJ, et al. Anterior cruciate ligament graft fixation. Initial comparison of patellar tendon and semitendinosus autografts in young fresh cadavers. Am J Sports Med 1997;25:472–8.

32. Woo SL, Hollis JM, Adams DJ, et al. Tensile properties of the human femur-anterior cruciate ligament-tibia complex. The effects of specimen age and orientation. Am J Sports Med 1991;19:217–25.

33. Cooper DE, Deng XH, Burstein AL, et al. The strength of the central third patellar tendon graft. A biomechanical study. Am J Sports Med 1993;21:818–23.

34. To JT, Howell SM, Hull ML. Contributions of femoral fixation methods to the stiffness of anterior cruciate ligament replacements at implantation. Arthroscopy 1999;15: 379–87.

35. Hamner DL, Brown CH Jr, Steiner ME, et al. Hamstring tendon grafts for reconstruction of the anterior cruciate ligament: biomechanical evaluation of the use of multiple strands and tensioning techniques. J Bone Joint Surg Am 1999;81:549–57.

36. Beynnon BD, Johnson RJ, Fleming BC, et al. Anterior cruciate ligament replacement: comparison of bone–patellar tendon–bone grafts with two-strand hamstring grafts. A prospective, randomized study. J Bone Joint Surg Am 2002;84-A(9):1503–13.

37. Pinczewski LA, Deehan DJ, Salmon LJ, et al. A five-year comparison of patellar tendon versus four-strand hamstring tendon autograft for arthroscopic reconstruction of the anterior cruciate ligament. Am J Sports Med 2002;30:523–36.

38. Harilainen A, Linko E, Sandelin J. Randomized prospective study of ACL reconstruction with interference screw fixation in patellar tendon autografts versus femoral metal plate suspension and tibial post fixation in hamstring tendon autografts: 5-year clinical and radiological follow-up results. Knee Surg Sports Traumatol Arthrosc 2006;14(6): 517–28.

39. Tow BP, Chang PC, Mitra AK, et al. Comparing 2-year outcomes of anterior cruciate ligament reconstruction using either patella-tendon or semitendinosus-tendon autografts: a non-randomised prospective study. J Orthop Surg (Hong Kong) 2005; 13(2):139–46.

40. Laxdal G, Kartus J, Hansson L, et al. A prospective randomized comparison of bone-patellar tendon-bone and hamstring grafts for anterior cruciate ligament reconstruction. Arthroscopy 2005;21(1):34–42.

41. Ejerhed L, Kartus J, Sernert N, et al. Patellar tendon or semitendinosus tendon autografts for anterior cruciate ligament reconstruction? A prospective randomized study with a two-year follow-up. Am J Sports Med 2003;31:19–25.

42. Jansson KA, Linko E, Sandelin J, et al. A prospective randomized study of patellar versus hamstring tendon autografts for anterior cruciate ligament reconstruction. Am J Sports Med. 2003;31(1):12–8.

43. Sajovic M, Vengust V, Komadina R, et al. A prospective, randomized comparison of semitendinosus and gracilis tendon versus patellar tendon autografts for anterior cruciate ligament reconstruction: five-year follow-up. Am J Sports Med 2006;34(12): 1933–40. Epub 2006 Aug 21.

44. Hadjicostas PT, Soucacos PN, Paessler HH, et al. Morphologic and histologic comparison between the patella and hamstring tendons grafts: a descriptive and anatomic study. Arthroscopy 2007;23(7):751–6.

45. Amiel D, Kleiner JB, Roux RD, et al. The phenomenon of "ligamentization": anterior cruciate ligament reconstruction with autogenous patellar tendon. J Orthop Res 1986;4:162–72.

46. Arnoczky SP, Tarvin GB, Marshall JL. Anterior cruciate ligament replacement using patellar tendon. An evaluation of graft revascularization in the dog. J Bone Joint Surg Am 1982;64:217–24.

47. Rougraff B, Shelbourne KD, Gerth PK, et al. Arthroscopic and histologic analysis of human patellar tendon autografts used for anterior cruciate ligament reconstruction. Am J Sports Med 1993;21:277–84.

48. Goradia VK, Rochat MC, Kida M, et al. Natural history of a hamstring tendon autograft used for anterior cruciate ligament reconstruction in a sheep model. Am J Sports Med 2000;28:40–6.

49. Lane JG, McFadden P, Bowden K, et al. The ligamentization process: a 4 year case study following ACL reconstruction with a semitendinosis graft. Arthroscopy 1993;9: 149–53.

50. Kartus J, Magnusson L, Stener S, et al. Complications following arthroscopic anterior cruciate ligament reconstruction. A 2-5-year follow-up of 604 patients with special emphasis on anterior knee pain. Knee Surg Sports Traumatol Arthrosc 1999;7:2–8.

51. Järvela T, Kannus P, Järvinen M. Anterior knee pain 7 years after an anterior cruciate ligament reconstruction with a bone–patellar tendon–bone autograft. Scand J Med Sci Sports 2000;10:221–7.

52. Shelbourne KD, Trumper RV. Preventing anterior knee pain after anterior cruciate ligament reconstruction. Am J Sports Med 1997;25:41–7.

53. Eriksson K, Anderberg P, Hamberg P, et al. A comparison of quadruple semitendinosus and patellar tendon grafts in reconstruction of the anterior cruciate ligament. J Bone Joint Surg Br 2001;83(3):348–54.

54. Corry IS, Webb JM, Clingeleffer AJ, et al. Arthroscopic reconstruction of the anterior cruciate ligament. A comparison of patellar tendon autograft and four-strand hamstring tendon autograft. Am J Sports Med 1999;27:444–54.

55. Otto D, Pinczewski LA, Clingeleffer A, et al. Five-year results of single-incision arthroscopic anterior cruciate ligament reconstruction with patellar tendon autograft. Am J Sports Med 1998;26:181–8.

56. Sachs RA, Daniel DM, Stone ML, et al. Patellofemoral problems after anterior cruciate ligament reconstruction. Am J Sports Med 1989;17:760–5.

57. Bonamo JJ, Krinick RM, Sporn AA. Rupture of the patellar ligament after use of its central third for anterior cruciate reconstruction. A report of two cases. J Bone Joint Surg Am 1984;66:1294–7.

58. Langan P, Fontanetta AP. Rupture of the patellar tendon after use of its central third. Orthop Rev 1987;16:317–21.

59. Piva SR, Childs JD, Klucinec BM, et al. Patella fracture during rehabilitation after bone-patellar tendon-bone anterior cruciate ligament reconstruction: 2 case reports. Orthop Sports Phys Ther 2009;39(4):278–86.

60. Brownstein B, Bronner S. Patella fractures associated with accelerated ACL rehabilitation in patients with autogenous patella tendon reconstructions. J Orthop Sports Phys Ther 1997;26(3):168–72.

61. Viola R, Vianello R. Three cases of patella fracture in 1,320 anterior cruciate ligament reconstructions with bone-patellar tendon-bone autograft. Arthroscopy 1999;15(1):93–7.

62. Voos JE, Drakos MC, Lorich DG, et al. Proximal tibia fracture after anterior cruciate ligament reconstruction using bone-patellar tendon-bone autograft: a case report. HSS J 2008;4(1):20–4.

63. Viola RW, Sterett WI, Newfield D, et al. Internal and external tibial rotation strength after anterior cruciate ligament reconstruction using ipsilateral semitendinosus and gracilis tendon autografts. Am J Sports Med 2000;28:552–5.

64. Segawa H, Omori G, Koga Y, et al. Rotational muscle strength of the limb after anterior cruciate ligament reconstruction using semitendinosus and gracilis tendon. Arthroscopy 2002;18:177–82.

65. Gobbi A. Single versus double hamstring tendon harvest for ACL reconstruction. Sports Med Arthrosc 2010;18(1):15–9.

Pediatric Anterior Cruciate Ligament Reconstruction with Autograft or Allograft

James L. Carey, MD, MPH[a,b,]*

KEYWORDS

• Anterior cruciate ligament • Autograft • Allograft • Pediatric

Anterior cruciate ligament (ACL) reconstruction in the pediatric population can be performed with the use of either autograft or allograft tissue. Commonly used autograft tissues include bone-patellar tendon-bone, hamstring tendons, and quadriceps tendon. Similarly, commonly used allograft tissues include bone-patellar tendon-bone, hamstring tendons, Achilles tendon, and tibialis tendons.

Reconstruction with autograft tissue has been the gold-standard procedure. In the clinical setting, the patient knows where this tissue has been for the entire life of the graft. For example, a 14-year-old girl knows that the ACL reconstruction will use her 14-year old tendon. However, there are potential drawbacks with harvesting this tissue, including increased pain in the immediate postoperative period and long-term sequellae, such as kneeling pain for bone-tendon-bone procedures or potential loss of flexion strength hamstring procedures.

Reconstruction with allograft tissue has advantages including the fact that it eliminates this donor-site morbidity. In this setting, however, the patient knows little about the origins of the tissue. The same 14-year-old girl may have an ACL reconstruction using a graft from a 14-year-old girl or a tendon from a 40-year-old man or woman. Although screening mechanisms exist, reconstruction with allograft tissue has the disadvantage of potentially transmitting diseases, including bacteria and viruses. In addition, there are concerns of slower incorporation and less robust healing.

The primary purpose of the current review is to determine if the short-term failure rates of ACL reconstruction with allograft are significantly different from those with autograft in the pediatric population. A secondary purpose is to review some special

The author has nothing to disclose.

[a] Department of Orthopaedic Surgery, University of Pennsylvania, 3400 Spruce Street, 2 Silverstein, Philadelphia, PA 19104, USA

[b] Penn Center for Advanced Cartilage Repair and Osteochondritis Dissecans Treatment, Weightman Hall, 235 South 33rd Street, Philadelphia, PA 19104, USA

* Penn Center for Advanced Cartilage Repair and Osteochondritis Dissecans Treatment, Weightman Hall, 235 South 33rd Street, Philadelphia, PA 19104.

E-mail address: james.carey@vanderbilt.edu

Clin Sports Med 30 (2011) 759–766

doi:10.1016/j.csm.2011.06.002

sportsmed.theclinics.com

considerations regarding graft choice that may be incorporated into the informed-consent and shared decision-making process.

COMPARATIVE STUDIES REPORTING CLINICAL OUTCOMES
All Ages—Previous Work

A systematic review and meta-analysis recently investigated whether the short-term clinical outcomes of ACL reconstruction with allograft were significantly different from those with autograft.[1] That systematic review process began with a computerized search of the electronic databases MEDLINE (from 1950 to the fourth week of March 2009) and EMBASE (from 1966 to March 2009), using the 3 keywords in combination: "auto$," "allo$," and "anterior cruciate ligament."[1] A study had to be a therapeutic study with a prospective or retrospective comparative design (level of evidence I, II, or III)[2] in order to be included.[1] In addition, each study had to compare autograft with allograft with use of the same anatomic graft and have a minimum duration of follow-up of 2 years.[1] Nine studies were included.[3-11]

That systematic review and meta-analysis found that the short-term clinical outcomes (such as instrumented laxity and failure rate) of ACL reconstruction with allograft were not significantly different from those with autograft.[1] "However, it is important to note that none of these non-randomized studies stratified outcomes according to age or utilized multivariable modeling to mathematically control for age (or any other possible confounder, such as activity level, that is not equally distributed in the two treatment groups)."[1]

All Ages—Current Update

For the current review, an updated literature search was performed to augment the findings of the prior systematic review. Specifically, a computerized search of the electronic database MEDLINE (from the fourth week of March 2009 to the third week of January 2011) was performed, using the 3 keywords in combination: "auto$," "allo$," and "anterior cruciate ligament." This update found 39 articles. After using the same inclusion criteria from the prior systematic review (outlined above), 2 additional articles were included.[12,13]

Therefore, 11 studies were determined to be appropriate for the current review (Table 1).[3-13] Of note, failures were not identically defined in these 11 studies. The criteria for clinical failure included the following: subsequent revision ACL reconstruction[3,5,8,10]; traumatic graft rupture[4,9,11]; positive Lachman testing with complaints of instability[9]; a side-to-side difference of greater than 5 mm on arthrometer testing[12]; and a combination of positive Lachman testing, positive pivot-shift testing, and a side-to-side difference of greater than 5 mm on arthrometer testing.[3,10] If clinical failure was not distinctly defined,[7,13] then the side-to-side difference of greater than 5 mm on arthrometer testing was used.

Interestingly, both of the additional studies were randomized controlled trials that shared the same 6 authors.[12,13] The first article documented the treatment of 172 patients undergoing ACL reconstruction with bone-patellar tendon-bone between May 2000 and June 2004 who were prospectively randomized into autograft or nonirradiated allograft groups.[13] The second article documented the treatment of 99 patients undergoing ACL reconstruction with bone-patellar tendon-bone between July 2004 and June 2006 who were prospectively randomized into autograft, nonirradiated allograft, and irradiated allograft (2.5 megarad) groups.[12]

These 2 randomized controlled trials[12,13] are substantially less susceptible to bias compared with the study designs of the other 9 included studies,[3-11] which were nonrandomized prospective and retrospective studies. Randomization eliminates the

Table 1
Selected study characteristics and clinical outcomes

First Author	Journal	Year	Level of Evidence	Patient Age (yr)	Follow-up Patients	Follow-up Time (mo)	Graft Type	Sterilization Method	Autograft (%)	Allograft (%)	P Value
				Study Characteristics					Failures		
Barrett	Am J Sports Med	2005	III	46 (40–58)	63	41 (24–99)	BPTB	Nonirradiated	0/25 (0%)	1/38 (3%)	NS
Chang	Arthroscopy	2003	III	31 (13–52)	79	37 (24–56)	BPTB	30 nonirradiated[a] 10 irradiated (dose unknown)	0/33 (0%)	3/46 (7%)	.1
Edgar	Clin Orthop Relat Res	2008	II	29	83	50 (36–70)	Hamstring (quadruple)	Nonirradiated	3/37 (8%)	2/46 (4%)	NS
Gorschewsky	Am J Sports Med	2005	II	NR	186	71 (54–80)	BPTB	Acetone solvent drying; irradiation (1.5 Mrad)	6/101 (6%)	38/85 (45%)	.005
Harner	Clin Orthop Relat Res	1996	III	24	90	45 (30–75)	BPTB[b]	Nonirradiated	2/26 (8%)	4/64 (6%)	NS
Kleipool	Knee Surg Sports Traumatol Arthrosc	1998	II	28 (14–43)	62	49 (30–74)	BPTB	Nonirradiated	0/26 (0%)	0/36 (0%)	NS
Peterson	Arthroscopy	2001	II	27 (15–55)	60	63 (55–78)	BPTB	Nonirradiated	1/30 (3%)	1/30 (3%)	NS

(continued on next page)

Table 1
(continued)

First Author	Journal	Year	Level of Evidence	Patient Age (yr)	Follow-up Patients	Follow-up Time (mo)	Graft Type	Sterilization Method	Autograft (%)	Allograft (%)	P Value
										Failures	
			Study Characteristics								
Saddemi	Arthroscopy	1993	III	22	50	24	BPTB	Irradiated (2.0 Mrad)	1/31 (3%)	1/19 (5%)	NS
Sun	Arthroscopy	2009	I	32 (19–65)	156	67 (48–96)	BPTB	Nonirradiated	5/76 (7%)	6/80 (8%)	NS
Sun	Knee Surg Sports Traumatol Arthrosc	2009	I	31 (16–64)	99	31 (24–47)	BPTB	34 nonirradiated 32 irradiated (2.5 Mrad)	**2/33 (6%)**	3/34 (9%) **11/32 (34%)**	NS **.011**
Victor	Int Orthop	1997	II	28 (18–43)	73	24	BPTB	NR	0/48 (0%)	3/25 (12%)	NR

Boldface signifies statistically significant difference.
Abbreviations: BPTB, Bone-patellar tendon-bone; NR, not reported; NS, not statistically significant; Mrad, megarad.
[a] Data on allograft preparation were only available for 40 of the 46 cases.
[b] For allografts, graft type was 60 BPTB and 4 Achilles.

Table 2
Autograft considerations

Advantages	Disadvantages
Known source and age of graft	Donor-site morbidity (bone-patellar tendon-bone)
No risk of disease transmission	Long-term kneeling pain
Gold-standard for healing	Risk of patellar fracture
Graft typically size-matched for ACL reconstruction	Donor-site morbidity (hamstrings)
Possible regeneration of tissue (central patellar tendon or hamstrings) after harvest	Long-term knee flexor strength deficit
	Risk of saphenous nerve trauma

selection bias introduced by the determination of treatment on the basis of patient choice. Combining the autograft and nonirradiated data from these 2 studies,[12,13] there were 7 failures out of 109 ACL reconstructions (6%) with autograft and 9 failures out of 104 ACL reconstructions (9%) with nonirradiated allograft, which was not a statistically significant difference. In contrast, there were 11 failures out of 32 ACL reconstructions (34%) with irradiated allograft.[12] The difference between failures in the autograft group and the irradiated allograft group was statistically significant ($P = .011$).

Pediatric Population

The mean age of the patients in these 11 studies was 30 years old, with a range of 13 to 65. Again, none of these studies stratified outcomes by age. Consequently, it is unclear if the failures are distributed evenly across the age and activity spectrum or are focused on a small number of athletes under age 16. Drawing conclusions about the relationships between graft choice and clinical outcome in the pediatric population (or any specific population, such as elite athletes) from aggregate data may be misleading because of biological or statistical interaction from interdependent operation of these factors, such as age, activity level, and graft choice.

SPECIAL CONSIDERATIONS IN THE PEDIATRIC POPULATION

There are several advantages and disadvantages to undergoing ACL reconstruction with autograft tissue (**Table 2**) or with allograft tissue (**Table 3**). In addition to overall clinical outcomes (detailed above), the patient must primarily consider a balance between possible long-term donor-site morbidity with autograft and possible disease transmission with allograft.

Autograft Long-term Donor-site Morbidity

Although patients appreciate that harvesting autograft bone-patellar tendon-bone will result in more pain in the immediate postoperative period, they often wish to understand the risk of long-term anterior knee pain. A recently conducted systematic review analyzed the intermediate-term outcomes (minimum of 5 years after ACL reconstruction) by graft type, comparing autograft bone-patellar tendon-bone with autograft hamstring tendons.[14] Interestingly, there was no appreciable difference in overall clinical outcomes between these 2 groups.[14] However, kneeling pain was consistently worse in the reconstruction group with autograft bone-patellar tendon-bone.[14] Therefore, autograft bone-patellar tendon-bone may be a suboptimal

Table 3
Allograft considerations

Advantages	Disadvantages
No donor-site morbidity	Potential for disease transmission
Shorter operative time	Variable procurement and processing
Less postoperative pain	Possible slower graft incorporation
Improved cosmesis	Limited availability
Cost of graft	Increased failure rates associated with certain sterilization methods, including irradiation
Allows for multiple grafts for multiligamentous reconstructions	

option for a child whose recreation or religion requires repetitive kneeling. Of note, another consideration in using autograft bone-patellar tendon-bone in a child is the skeletal maturity of the tibial tubercle. If the tibial tubercle is nearly skeletally mature, then the bone plugs should be carefully fashioned to readily slide through the bony tunnels with minimal resistance, and the main traction sutures for pulling the graft should be placed in the patellar plug rather than in the tibial plug.

Similarly, although patients appreciate that harvesting a subset of their 4 hamstring tendons will result in less hamstring strength in the immediate postoperative period, they often wish to understand the risk of long-term knee flexor strength deficits. A recent study compared the mean peak isometric knee flexor torque of the following 3 groups: subjects 2 years after ACL reconstruction using autograft hamstring tendons (semitendinosus-gracilis); subjects 2 years after ACL reconstruction using allograft tibialis anterior tendons; and a noninjured, activity-level–matched control group.[15] Again, the 2 ACL reconstructed groups did not differ in clinical outcomes.[15] However, the group that underwent reconstruction with autograft hamstring tendons demonstrated a lower peak isometric knee flexor torque compared with the other groups (~23% lower, $P<.05$).[15] Therefore, autograft hamstring tendons may be a suboptimal choice in a child whose recreation requires sprinting or hurdling.

Allograft Potential for Disease Transmission

Allograft tissue used in ACL reconstruction has been reported as a source of viral and bacterial infections. Specifically, a case of acute hepatitis C transmission[16] as well as a case of human immunodeficiency virus (HIV) transmission[17] have been reported in patients who underwent ACL reconstruction with allograft bone-patellar tendon-bone. In addition, there have been several reports of isolated cases and clusters of bacterial infections related to ACL reconstruction with contaminated allograft tissue.[18–21]

There is a risk benefit ratio to irradiation treatment for grafts, in that irradiation of viral particles and bacteria may eliminate infectivity,[17] but certain levels of irradiation may also cause structural damage to the graft, which can increase the failure rate.[12] Consequently, donor screening is the primary means of preventing transmission of viral infections,[16] and a time window exists between initial infection with a virus and the ability to detect the presence of the virus or its antibody response on a screening panel.[16]

COST

Although arriving at a graft choice is a medical decision primarily involving the child, the child's family, and the surgeon, the cost of these options ultimately affects their availability in certain settings. Two studies have analyzed the cost of ACL reconstruction with autograft and allograft tissue.[22,23] In the setting of all procedures performed in an outpatient setting, ACL reconstruction with allograft (US $5465) was more costly than ACL reconstruction with autograft (US $4872). In contrast, if the increased pain from autograft harvest sometimes resulted in hospitalization, then ACL reconstruction with autograft (US $5694) was more costly than ACL reconstruction with allograft (US $4622).[23] Increased operating room time and a greater likelihood of overnight hospitalization at some facilities increase the cost of ACL reconstruction with autograft.[23] The cost of operating room supplies (primarily the allograft itself) increases the cost of ACL reconstruction with allograft.[23]

SUMMARY

The surgeon may include the following key points into the informed-consent and shared-decision–making process to individualize optimum patient care:

1) The short-term outcomes of ACL reconstruction with nonirradiated allograft tissue are not significantly different from those with autograft tissue. Failure rates with irradiated allograft tissue, however, are significantly higher.
2) Potential long-term donor site morbidity includes kneeling pain after harvest of autograft bone-patellar tendon-bone and knee flexor strength deficits after harvest of autograft hamstring tendons.
3) The risk of viral and bacterial transmission from allograft tissue is very low, and careful donor screening and aseptic processing minimize but do not completely eliminate this risk.

REFERENCES

1. Carey JL, Dunn WR, Dahm DL, et al. A systematic review of anterior cruciate ligament reconstruction with autograft compared with allograft. J Bone Joint Surg Am 2009; 91(9):2242–50.
2. Wright JG, Swiontkowski MF, Heckman JD. Introducing levels of evidence to the journal. J Bone Joint Surg Am 2003;85-A(1):1–3.
3. Barrett G, Stokes D, White M. Anterior cruciate ligament reconstruction in patients older than 40 years: allograft versus autograft patellar tendon. Am J Sports Med 2005;33(10):1505–12.
4. Chang SK, Egami DK, Shaieb MD, et al. Anterior cruciate ligament reconstruction: allograft versus autograft. Arthroscopy 2003;19(5):453–62.
5. Edgar CM, Zimmer S, Kakar S, et al. Prospective comparison of auto and allograft hamstring tendon constructs for ACL reconstruction. Clin Orthop Relat Res 2008; 466(9):2238–46.
6. Gorschewsky O, Klakow A, Riechert K, et al. Clinical comparison of the Tutoplast allograft and autologous patellar tendon (bone-patellar tendon-bone) for the reconstruction of the anterior cruciate ligament: 2- and 6-year results. Am J Sports Med 2005;33(8):1202–9.
7. Harner CD, Olson E, Irrgang JJ, et al. Allograft versus autograft anterior cruciate ligament reconstruction: 3- to 5-year outcome. Clin Orthop Relat Res 1996(324):134–44.

8. Kleipool AE, Zijl JA, Willems WJ. Arthroscopic anterior cruciate ligament reconstruction with bone-patellar tendon-bone allograft or autograft. A prospective study with an average follow up of 4 years. Knee Surg Sports Traumatol Arthrosc 1998;6(4):224–30.

9. Peterson RK, Shelton WR, Bomboy AL. Allograft versus autograft patellar tendon anterior cruciate ligament reconstruction: a 5-year follow-up. Arthroscopy 2001;17(1): 9–13.

10. Saddemi SR, Frogameni AD, Fenton PJ, et al. Comparison of perioperative morbidity of anterior cruciate ligament autografts versus allografts. Arthroscopy 1993;9(5):519–24.

11. Victor J, Bellemans J, Witvrouw E, et al. Graft selection in anterior cruciate ligament reconstruction—prospective analysis of patellar tendon autografts compared with allografts. Int Orthop 1997;21(2):93–7.

12. Sun K, Tian S, Zhang J, et al. Anterior cruciate ligament reconstruction with BPTB autograft, irradiated versus non-irradiated allograft: a prospective randomized clinical study. Knee Surg Sports Traumatol Arthrosc 2009;17(5):464–74.

13. Sun K, Tian SQ, Zhang JH, et al. Anterior cruciate ligament reconstruction with bone-patellar tendon-bone autograft versus allograft. Arthroscopy 2009;25(7): 750–9.

14. Magnussen RA, Carey JL, Spindler KP. Does autograft choice determine intermediate-term outcome of ACL reconstruction? Knee Surg Sports Traumatol Arthrosc 2011;19:462–72.

15. Landes S, Nyland J, Elmlinger B, et al. Knee flexor strength after ACL reconstruction: comparison between hamstring autograft, tibialis anterior allograft, and non-injured controls. Knee Surg Sports Traumatol Arthrosc 2010;18(3):317–24.

16. CDC. Hepatitis C virus transmission from an antibody-negative organ and tissue donor—United States, 2000–2002. MMWR Morb Mortal Wkly Rep 2003;52(13): 273–6.

17. Asselmeier MA, Caspari RB, Bottenfield S. A review of allograft processing and sterilization techniques and their role in transmission of the human immunodeficiency virus. Am J Sports Med 1993;21(2):170–5.

18. CDC. Septic arthritis following anterior cruciate ligament reconstruction using tendon allografts—Florida and Louisiana, 2000. MMWR Morb Mortal Wkly Rep 2001;50(48): 1081–3.

19. Crawford C, Kainer M, Jernigan D, et al. Investigation of postoperative allograft-associated infections in patients who underwent musculoskeletal allograft implantation. Clin Infect Dis 2005;41(2):195–200.

20. CDC. Invasive streptococcus pyogenes after allograft implantation—Colorado, 2003. MMWR Morb Mortal Wkly Rep 2003;52(48):1173–6.

21. CDC. Update: allograft-associated bacterial infections—United States, 2002. MMWR Morb Mortal Wkly Rep 2002;51(10):207–10.

22. Nagda SH, Altobelli GG, Bowdry KA, et al. Cost analysis of outpatient anterior cruciate ligament reconstruction: autograft versus allograft. Clin Orthop Relat Res 2010; 468(5):1418–22.

23. Cole DW, Ginn TA, Chen GJ, et al. Cost comparison of anterior cruciate ligament reconstruction: autograft versus allograft. Arthroscopy 2005;21(7):786–90.

Physeal-Sparing Anterior Cruciate Ligament Reconstruction with Iliotibial Band

Anne Marie Chicorell, DO, MPH[a], Adam Y. Nasreddine, MA[b],
Mininder S. Kocher, MD, MPH[c,d],*

KEYWORDS

- Iliotibial band • Skeletally immature • Physeal sparing
- Anterior cruciate ligament

The knee is the most common site of injury in the skeletally immature athlete.[1] Recent estimates prove that 6.7% of total anterior cruciate ligament (ACL) injuries and 30.8% of youth knee injuries occur in the pediatric population.[2] There are controversies as to whether ACL injuries are truly on the rise because of increased participation and demands at a younger age or if it is a combination of heightened awareness and increased diagnostic imagery. Treatment of ACL injuries within this subpopulation is controversial as well. Whereas operative treatment places risk to the physis, nonoperative management may lead to functional instability, which predisposes the athlete to potential meniscal and/or chondral damage. Surgeons must also consider skeletal maturity, physiologic age, desired goals, patient compliance, associated injuries, and relative surgical risk. By performing physeal-sparing intraarticular and extraarticular iliotibial (IT) band reconstruction of the ACL, risk of physeal injury is reduced and stability of the knee is restored. This article reviews the indications for IT band reconstruction of the ACL in the skeletally immature athlete, surgical technique, pitfalls, and results of treatment.

BIOLOGICAL CONSIDERATIONS

The patient's physiologic age and growth potential are important in choosing the appropriate surgical procedure for ACL reconstruction. Radiographs and developmental findings are used to determine the physiologic age. Referencing

The authors have nothing to disclose. None did receive any financial support pertaining to this work.
[a] Division of Sports Medicine, Department of Orthopaedic Surgery, Children's Hospital Boston, 319 Longwood Avenue, Boston, MA 02115, USA
[b] Department of Orthopaedic Surgery, Children's Hospital Boston, Fegan 134, 300 Longwood Avenue, Boston, MA 02115, USA
[c] Division of Sports Medicine, Children's Hospital Boston, Boston, MA, USA
[d] Harvard Medical School, 300 Longwood Avenue, Hunnewell 2, Boston, MA 02115, USA
* Corresponding author. Harvard Medical School, 300 Longwood Avenue, Hunnewell 2, Boston, MA 02115.
E-mail address: mininder.kocher@childrens.harvard.edu

Clin Sports Med 30 (2011) 767–777
doi:10.1016/j.csm.2011.07.005
0278-5919/11/$ – see front matter © 2011 Elsevier Inc. All rights reserved.

Table 1
Tanner staging classification of secondary sexual characteristics

Tanner Stage		Boy	Girl
Stage 1 (Prepubertal)	Growth	5–6 cm/y	5–6 cm/y
	Development	Testes < 4 mL or < 2.5 cm	No breast development
		No pubic hair	No pubic hair
Stage 2	Growth	5–6 cm/y	7–8 cm/y
	Development	Testes 4 mL or 2.5–3.2 cm	Breast buds
		Minimal pubic hair at base of penis	Minimal pubic hair on labia
Stage 3	Growth	7–8 cm/y	8 cm/y
	Development	Testes 12 mL or 3.6 cm	Elevation of breast; areolae enlarge
		Pubic hair over pubis	Pubic hair of mons pubis
		Voice changes	Axillary hair
		Muscle mass increases	Acne
Stage 4	Growth	10 cm/y	7 cm/y
	Development	Testes 4.1–4.5 cm	Areolae enlarge
		Pubic hair as adult	Pubic hair as adult
		Axillary hair	
		Acne	
Stage 5	Growth	No growth	No growth
	Development	Testes as adult	Adult breast contour
		Pubic hair as adult	Pubic hair as adult
		Facial hair as adult	
		Mature physique	
Other		Peak Height Velocity: 13.5 y	Adrenarche: 6–8 y
			Menarche 12.7 y
			Peak Height Velocity: 11.5 y

radiographs of the left wrist to the atlas of Greulich and Pyle provides an efficient means to determine skeletal age preoperatively. The physiologic age is based on the Tanner staging system[3] (**Table 1**).

During puberty, advances in coordination, strength, and endurance may vary. The growth spurt begins at age 9 for girls and 11 for boys, and may contribute around 20% of a child's total adult height. Girls may have between 2.5 and 3 inches of growth remaining postmenarche. Peak height velocity for girls occurs at age 11 to 12 (2.5–4.5 in/y), Tanner 2, whereas boys are a little older from 13 to 14 (3–5 in/y), Tanner 4.

ANATOMIC CONSIDERATIONS

The choice of surgical technique is dependent on the physiologic age of the patient and the amount of growth remaining (**Fig. 1**). Distal femur growth accounts for 71%

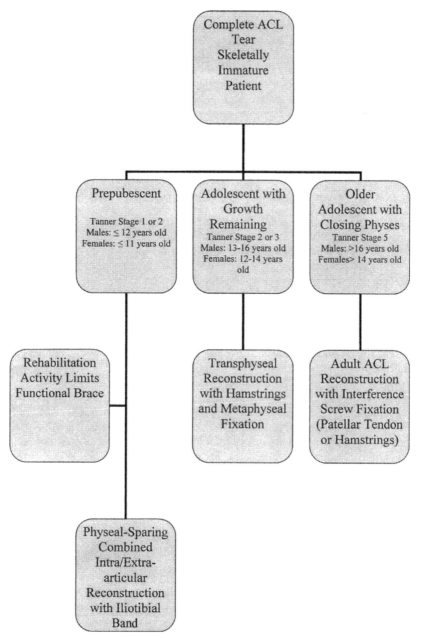

Fig. 1. Algorithm for management of complete ACL injuries in skeletally immature patients.

of the total femur growth and 37% of the entire lower limb growth at a rate of about 1.2 cm/yr. The proximal tibia accounts for 57% of the total tibial growth and 28% of the entire lower limb growth at a rate of about 0.9 cm/yr. This information is critical in ACL surgery because the knee then accounts for two-thirds of the lower extremity growth potential.[4–6]

The prepubescent child (Tanner stage 1 or 2) with a midsubstance ACL tear presents a difficult problem. Because of the large amount of growth remaining, the consequences of iatrogenic physeal arrest are severe. Unfortunately, activity modification such as refraining from cutting sports is difficult in this age group, and nonreconstructive treatment has been associated with meniscal and chondral injury.[7–10]

For prepubescent children, violation of the tibial and femoral physis presents a risk of growth disturbance that could require limb lengthening or osteotomy. Animal studies have demonstrated a risk of physeal arrest with transphyseal ACL reconstruction.[11–13] Several clinical reports have documented growth disturbances following ACL reconstruction in this age group.[14–16] Possible factors contributing to growth disturbance are size of drill hole, graft placement, hardware placement, and graft tension.[11,12,17,18]

HISTORY AND PHYSICAL EXAMINATION FINDINGS

The initial evaluation by the practitioner is invaluable in developing a differential diagnosis and determining appropriate treatment. The history should include the mechanism of injury, instability, catching or locking, and an audible popping noise with subsequent effusion. The patient should also be asked about parental height, timing of growth spurt, and menarche (in girls). Midsubstance ACL ruptures are usually caused by a rapid deceleration and twisting mechanism and are diagnosed more frequently in pediatric athletes participating in cutting and contact sports. However, approximately two-thirds of ACL injuries occur by noncontact mechanisms.[19]

The findings on physical examination are dependent on the timing in relation to the injury. The Lachman test and pivot shift test are positive before swelling and guarding occurs. Rates of ACL injury are reported between 10% and 65% in pediatric patients presenting with traumatic hemarthrosis of the knee; therefore, young athletes presenting with a hemarthrosis of the knee should raise suspicion for an ACL tear.[20–24] The differential diagnosis of hemarthrosis of the knee includes patellar dislocation, meniscal tear, osteochondral fracture, tibial spine fracture, and epiphyseal fracture of the femur or tibia.

A thorough examination of the knee must be performed to rule out concomitant injuries. Associated injuries include meniscal tears, posterior cruciate and/or collateral ligament tears, osteochondral fractures, and physeal fractures of the distal femur or proximal tibia. Given the higher prevalence of generalized ligamentous laxity in skeletally immature patients, a direct comparison with the contralateral knee should also be made.

IMAGING

Initial radiographs should include anteroposterior, lateral, notch, and sunrise views to rule out a tibial spine fracture or patella dislocation. If a disruption of the ligament is suspected on clinical examination and radiographs are negative, then magnetic resonance imaging (MRI) is warranted. The knee can be further evaluated for bone contusion at the posterior lateral tibial plateau and lateral femoral condyle and for associated meniscal and ligament injuries. MRI is useful to distinguish between partial tears, avulsions, and midsubstance tears of the ACL as well.

INDICATIONS AND TIMING OF SURGERY

Indications for ACL reconstruction in a skeletally immature patient include complete ACL tear with functional instability, partial ACL tear that has failed nonoperative treatment, and ACL injury with associated repairable meniscal or chondral injury. Because of higher rates of postoperative stiffness, acute ACL reconstruction is not recommended for isolated ACL tears.[25] Surgery is typically delayed 3 weeks from the time of injury or until adequate range of motion has been achieved.

The natural history of ACL tears in the skeletally immature is similar to that of adults. Chronic instability leads to meniscal damage, chondral injury, and osteoarthritis. In the ACL-deficient knee, the posterior horn of the medial meniscus is the secondary restraint to anterior translation of tibia on femur. Forces increase by 57% in extension and 197% in flexion in an ACL-deficient knee. The incidence of associated injuries with ACL tears in the pediatric population was 58% in those with acute tears and 73% in those with chronic tears.[26] This incidence suggests that the longer patients are ACL deficient the more at risk they are for developing associated injuries, which is why the authors advocate reconstruction avoiding the growth plate.

TREATMENT OPTIONS

Surgical techniques include physeal sparing and transphyseal and partial transphyseal reconstructions. In theory the extraarticular reconstruction provides a method to restore stability and avoid risk of growth disturbance. Isolated extraarticular reconstructions in children have had variable long-term results. Nakhostine[27] reported on 5 patients with open growth plates who underwent anterior cruciate reconstruction with a strip of IT band placed over the top of the lateral femoral condyle in a MacIntosh-type repair. At 4.4-year follow-up, the patients reported subjective satisfaction and ability to return to sport. Clinically, 3 of the 5 had greater than or equal to a 3-mm side-to-side difference on KT-2000 testing and all the patients had a +2 Lachman test. In the survey of the Herodicus Society of management and complications of ACL injuries in skeletally immature patients there were 15 reported cases of growth disturbances with a large variance in fixation and surgical technique.[14,28] McCarroll[28] reported on results of 10 patients followed for 26 months with no growth disturbances. All returned to sports, but 4 had a single incidence of instability and 1 required revision ACL reconstruction and meniscal repair as an adolescent. At the authors' institution we use a modification of the MacIntosh ACL reconstruction to perform a physeal-sparing reconstruction with an extraarticular and intraarticular component. A portion of the IT band is harvested from the lateral thigh. The IT band remains attached to the proximal tibia at the Gerdy tubercle. The band is fixed to the proximal femur constituting the extraarticular portion of the reconstruction. The proximal portion of the IT band is then passed from the posterior aspect of the lateral femoral condyle through the intercondylar notch, under the intermeniscal ligament and fixed at the proximal tibial metaphysis to provide an intraarticular reconstruction. The results of 44 patients with a mean follow-up of 5.3 years were examined. There were 2 failures at 4.7 and 8.3 years and no episodes of growth disturbance. The mean International Knee Documentation Committee (IKDC) subjective knee score and Lysholm score were 96.7 and 95.7.[29]

Surgical treatment with conventional transphyseal tunnels has been described.[29,30] Liddle and colleagues[30] describe the results of 17 patients treated with transphyseal ACL reconstruction with four-strand hamstring autograft. Eight Tanner stage 1 and 9 Tanner stage 2 patients were followed for a mean of 44 months. The mean Lysholm score at follow-up was 97.5. There was one failure due to an additional injury. One child was noted to have a 5° valgus deformity.

An alternative physeal-sparing technique using epiphyseal tunnels has been described by Anderson.[31] A transepiphyseal technique using fluoroscopy was performed in 12 patients. The mean IKDC Subjective score was 96.4 at 4.1 years, with no graft failures or growth arrests noted. Another alternative is physeal sparing on the femoral side only and transtibial. The tibial drill holes are central and vertical with soft-tissue autograft, which prevents tibial impingement. This technique has proved to be efficacious with no evidence of leg length discrepancy or angular deformity noted if fixation or bone plug did not cross the physis.[32–34]

In a pediatric patient nearing skeletal maturity, nonphyseal-sparing transtibial and transfemoral reconstruction can be considered. The advantages to this technique are isometric graft position and reliable results, with the disadvantage of potential growth disturbance.[12,28, 35–41]

Mohtadi and Grant[42] performed a systematic review to compare surgical with nonsurgical treatment of ACL deficiency in pediatric populations and help provide guidelines for clinicians. Their synopsis was that both ACL injury and meniscal damage are independent risk factors for development of osteoarthritis. Their proposed algorithm advocated nonoperative ACL reconstruction, even in patients treated with meniscal tears treated arthroscopically, until further instability episodes or injuries occur.[42] In the authors' population of active children, in order to promote continued sports participation and reduce the risk of further injury to the knee, they advocate reconstruction of the ACL avoiding the growth plate.

SURGICAL TECHNIQUE:PHYSEAL-SPARING INTRAARTICULAR AND EXTRAARTICULAR ACL RECONSTRUCTION WITH ILIOTIBIAL BAND

For prepubescent children, Tanner 1 or 2, a physeal-sparing reconstruction is recommended.[43] Skeletal age is usually less than 14 in boys and less than 13 in girls. The patient is placed supine on the operating room table. Examination under anesthesia is performed to confirm Tanner staging and verify ACL insufficiency. The operative extremity is prepped and draped from the level of the foot to the level of a tourniquet placed at the thigh. It is important to place the tourniquet as proximally as possible in case a counterincision is necessary to assist in harvesting the IT band proximally. The insertion of the IT band on the tibia is palpated at the Gerdy tubercle. The incision runs obliquely from the lateral joint line to the superior border of the IT band. The tourniquet is not routinely inflated in order to prevent tethering of the IT band. The incision is then made, and self-retaining retractors are placed. Dissection is carried down to the level of the IT band. In young, thin patients the IT band may be quite superficial. The anterior and posterior borders of the IT band are defined (**Fig. 2**A). Posteriorly, the IT band blends with the lateral hamstrings, and harvesting too posteriorly would risk injury to the common peroneal nerve. A Cobb elevator is used to dissect the subcutaneous tissue away from the IT band along its course.

In order to harvest the IT tendon, a 15 blade is used to make an incision at the anterior border starting 2 cm above the Gerdy tubercle. A Kelly clamp is placed in this incision and pushed posteriorly until the intramuscular septum is palpated. The clamp is then passed through the posterior border of the IT band just above the intramuscular septum. The clamp is then spread in line with the fibers of the tendon to start the posterior split in the tendon. Adhesions to the underlying tissue are often present and should be released. A meniscotome is used to extend the two incisions proximally. Two parallel cuts are made with the meniscotome in line with the fibers of the tendon and continued as proximally as possible. The angled meniscotome is then used to transect the graft proximally (see **Fig. 2**B). If there is difficulty releasing the graft with the curved meniscotome, an accessory incision is made near the tourniquet.

The graft is tabularized, and a whip stitch is placed at its proximal end with No. 5 Ethibond. The tendon is carefully separated from the underlying joint capsule and lateral femoral condyle. The capsule in this area is thin, but an effort should be made

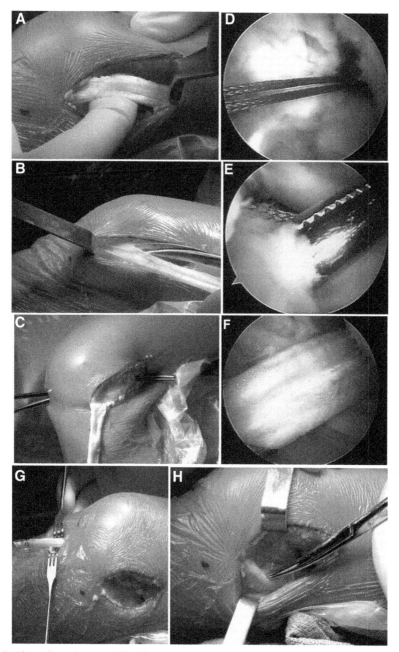

Fig. 2. Physeal-sparing, combined intraarticular, and extraarticular reconstruction using autogenous iliotibial band for prepubescents. (*A*) The graft is harvested through the lateral incision. (*B*) The graft is left attached to the Gerdy tubercle distally. (*C, D*) The graft is brought through the knee in the over-the-top position using a full-length clamp. (*E*) The graft is brought under the intermeniscal ligament. A groove can be made in the epiphysis in this region with a rasp. (*F*) Intraarticular reconstruction component. (*G*) The graft is brought out of the medial tibial incision and fixed here to a trough in the periosteum. (*H*) Extraarticular reconstruction component.

to maintain the integrity of the capsule to prevent fluid extravasation during later arthroscopy. The graft is separated distal to the femoral condyle so the tibia can be rotated with tension on the graft. This is the windlass effect and crucial for eliminating the pivot shift. The graft is left attached to the Gerdy tubercle distally and tucked under the skin for the arthroscopic portion of the case. The common pitfall is harvesting the IT band graft of inadequate length. To prevent this problem, use a longer incision or tendon stripper, or consider making an accessory incision proximally in the thigh.

A standard diagnostic arthroscopy is then performed. The leg is elevated and the tourniquet is inflated. The anterolateral viewing portal is established, and the arthroscope is inserted. An anteromedial portal is established under direct arthroscopic visualization. An arthroscopy is performed, and any associated injuries are treated. A limited notchplasty is used to aid in visualization and identification of the over-the-top position on the distal femur. Excessive dissection should be avoided to prevent injury to the perichondral ring of the distal femoral physis during notchplasty. The distance from the femoral footprint of the ACL to the physis is typically 3 to 5 mm.[44] Care is also taken to leave a portion of the native ACL and synovial tissue within the notch to act as an inferior sling to maintain the graft in the over-the-top position.

After dissection and visualization of the over-the-top position is complete, the IT band can be passed. A full-length clamp is placed through the anteromedial portal, through the notch, and into the over-the-top position. The clamp is then passed carefully through the joint capsule along the posterolateral femur and into the site of the IT band harvest (see **Fig. 2**C). It is important to maintain the clamp on the posterolateral femur during dissection to avoid neurovascular injury. Next a small nick is made just below the lateral intermuscular septum, which will later serve as the entry point for the IT band graft entering the over-the-top position. The clamp is visualized just below the lateral intermuscular septum and is then spread open to dilate a passage for the graft. The Ethibond sutures at the free end of the graft are placed into the clamp, and the graft is passed into the knee joint (see **Fig. 2**D).

The distal insertion of the graft is then prepared. An additional 3- to 5-cm incision is made on the anteromedial aspect of the proximal medial tibia in the region of the pes bursa. The incision must be distal to the tibial physis and medial to the tibial tubercle apophysis. Dissection is carried down to the periosteum. Under arthroscopic visualization a rasp is then passed along the periosteum and into the knee joint proximally. The rasp must enter the joint underneath the intermeniscal ligament. Using the rasp, a groove is then made in the tibial epiphysis in order to translate the graft posteriorly and achieve a more anatomic position. A clamp is placed through this groove, and the graft pulled under the intermeniscal ligament and delivered into the distal incision (see **Fig. 2**E).

Extraarticular fixation of the graft begins with femoral fixation. With the knee in 90° of flexion, tension is applied to the graft, and the proximal aspect of the graft is sutured to the periosteum of lateral femoral condyle and the lateral intermuscular septum (see **Fig. 2**G). This maneuver forms the extraarticular component of the reconstruction and helps to limit rotation of the tibia. Distally, an incision is made in the periosteum of the tibia. Periosteal flaps are raised medially and laterally with a cob in order to accommodate the diameter of the graft. Care is taken to avoid excessive medial dissection because this risks injury to the tibial tubercle apophysis. A trough is then created in the tibia using a burr or curettes. With the knee in 20° to 30° of flexion, distal tension is applied to the graft. No. 2 Fiberwire sutures are thrown from proximal to distal, then tied after all are placed. The authors use mattress sutures superficial to deep through the medial periosteum, medial to lateral through graft, then deep to superficial through lateral periosteum, angling the stitches proximally to increase graft tension when tied. At least three sutures should be placed proximally in the femur and distally in the tibia. Tibial fixation may be supplemented with a post if necessary.

Wounds are closed in layered fashion with absorbable suture with the knee in 15° of flexion. A sterile dressing and cryotherapy unit is then applied to the knee. Postoperative range of motion is limited from 0° to 30° for 2 weeks in both a hinged knee brace and a continuous passive motion unit. Flexion is increased to 90° from weeks 2 to 6, after which motion is unrestricted. Touchdown weightbearing in full extension is recommended for 6 weeks postoperatively. The patient may be placed into a simple hinge brace at 6 weeks; jogging is instituted at 3 months with return to cutting sports at 6 months pending clinical clearance. An ACL brace is worn for high-risk activities for the first 1 to 2 years after return to sport. Radiographs are obtained at 6 months to evaluate for physeal arrest. Clinical follow-up with assessment for leg length discrepancy or angular deformity is done yearly for at least 2 years. Additional radiographs are obtained as indicated by clinical examination.

REFERENCES

1. Smith AD, Tao SS. Knee injuries in young athletes. Clin Sports Med 1995;14:629–50.
2. Shea KG, Pfeiffer R, Wang JH, et al. Anterior cruciate ligament injury in pediatric and adolescent soccer players: an analysis of insurance data. J Pediatr Orthop 2004;24: 623–8.
3. Tanner JM, Whitehouse RH. Clinical longitudinal standards for height, weight, height velocity, weight velocity, and stages of puberty. Arch Dis Child 1976;51:170–9.
4. Anderson M, Green WT, Messner MB. Growth and predictions of growth in the lower extremities. J Bone Joint Surg Am 1963;45–A:1–14.
5. Pritchett JW. Longitudinal growth and growth-plate activity in the lower extremity. Clin Orthop Relat Res 1992:274–9.
6. Paley D, Bhave A, Herzenberg JE, et al. Multiplier method for predicting limb-length discrepancy. J Bone Joint Surg Am 2000;82–A:1432–46.
7. Andersson C, Odensten M, Good L, et al. Surgical or non-surgical treatment of acute rupture of the anterior cruciate ligament. A randomized study with long-term follow-up. J Bone Joint Surg Am 1989;71:965–74.
8. Giove TP, Miller SJ 3rd, Kent BE, et al. Non-operative treatment of the torn anterior cruciate ligament. J Bone Joint Surg Am 1983;65:184–92.
9. McDaniel WJ Jr, Dameron TB, Jr.The untreated anterior cruciate ligament rupture. Clin Orthop Relat Res 1983:158–63.
10. McDaniel WJ Jr, Dameron TB Jr. Untreated ruptures of the anterior cruciate ligament. A follow-up study. J Bone Joint Surg Am 1980;62:696–705.
11. Edwards TB, Greene CC, Baratta RV, et al. The effect of placing a tensioned graft across open growth plates. A gross and histologic analysis. J Bone Joint Surg Am 2001;83–A:725–34.
12. Guzzanti V, Falciglia F, Gigante A, et al. The effect of intra-articular ACL reconstruction on the growth plates of rabbits. J Bone Joint Surg Br 1994;76:960–3.
13. Houle JB, Letts M, Yang J. Effects of a tensioned tendon graft in a bone tunnel across the rabbit physis. Clin Orthop Relat Res 2001:275–81.
14. Kocher MS, Saxon HS, Hovis WD, et al. Management and complications of anterior cruciate ligament injuries in skeletally immature patients: survey of the Herodicus Society and The ACL Study Group. J Pediatr Orthop 2002;22:452–7.

15. Koman JD, Sanders JO. Valgus deformity after reconstruction of the anterior cruciate ligament in a skeletally immature patient. A case report. J Bone Joint Surg Am 1999;81:711–5.
16. Lipscomb AB, Anderson AF. Tears of the anterior cruciate ligament in adolescents. J Bone Joint Surg Am 1986;68:19–28.
17. Makela EA, Vainionpaa S, Vihtonen K, et al. The effect of trauma to the lower femoral epiphyseal plate. An experimental study in rabbits. J Bone Joint Surg Br 1988;70: 187–91.
18. Stadelmaier DM, Arnoczky SP, Dodds J, et al. The effect of drilling and soft tissue grafting across open growth plates. A histologic study. Am J Sports Med 1995;23: 431–5.
19. Noyes FR, Bassett RW, Grood ES, et al. Arthroscopy in acute traumatic hemarthrosis of the knee. Incidence of anterior cruciate tears and other injuries. J Bone Joint Surg Am 1980;62:687–95, 757.
20. Eiskjaer S, Larsen ST, Schmidt MB. The significance of hemarthrosis of the knee in children. Arch Orthop Trauma Surg 1988;107:96–8.
21. Kloeppel-Wirth S, Koltai JL, Dittmer H. Significance of arthroscopy in children with knee joint injuries. Eur J Pediatr Surg 1992;2:169–72.
22. Kocher MS, DiCanzio J, Zurakowski D, et al. Diagnostic performance of clinical examination and selective magnetic resonance imaging in the evaluation of intraarticular knee disorders in children and adolescents. Am J Sports Med 2001;29:292–6.
23. Luhmann SJ. Acute traumatic knee effusions in children and adolescents. J Pediatr Orthop 2003;23:199–202.
24. Vahasarja V, Kinnuen P, Serlo W. Arthroscopy of the acute traumatic knee in children. Prospective study of 138 cases. Acta Orthop Scand 1993;64:580–2.
25. Shelbourne KD, Wilckens JH, Mollabashy A, et al. Arthrofibrosis in acute anterior cruciate ligament reconstruction. The effect of timing of reconstruction and rehabilitation. Am J Sports Med 1991;19:332–6.
26. Millett PJ, Willis AA, Warren RF. Associated injuries in pediatric and adolescent anterior cruciate ligament tears: does a delay in treatment increase the risk of meniscal tear? Arthroscopy 2002;18:955–9.
27. Nakhostine M, Bollen SR, Cross MJ. Reconstruction of mid-substance anterior cruciate rupture in adolescents with open physes. J Pediatr Orthop 1995;15:286–7.
28. McCarroll JR, Rettig AC, Shelbourne KD. Anterior cruciate ligament injuries in the young athlete with open physes. Am J Sports Med 1988;16:44–7.
29. Anderson AF. Transepiphyseal replacement of the anterior cruciate ligament in skeletally immature patients. A preliminary report. J Bone Joint Surg Am 2003;85–A: 1255–63.
30. Liddle AD, Imbuldeniya AM, Hunt DM, et al. Transphyseal reconstruction of the anterior cruciate ligament in prepubescent children. J Bone Joint Surg Br 2008;90: 1317–22.
31. Anderson AF. Transepiphyseal replacement of the anterior cruciate ligament using quadruple hamstring grafts in skeletally immature patients. J Bone Joint Surg Am 2004;86–A Suppl 1:201–9.
32. Andrews JR, Sanders R. A "mini-reconstruction" technique in treating anterolateral rotatory instability (ALRI). Clin Orthop Relat Res 1983:93–6.
33. Lo IK, Bell DM, Fowler PJ. Anterior cruciate ligament injuries in the skeletally immature patient. Instr Course Lect 1998;47:351–9.
34. Bisson LJ, Wickiewicz T, Levinson M, et al. ACL reconstruction in children with open physes. Orthopedics 1998;21:659–63.

35. Aichroth PM, Patel DV, Zorrilla P. The natural history and treatment of rupture of the anterior cruciate ligament in children and adolescents. A prospective review. J Bone Joint Surg Br 2002;84:38–41.
36. Fuchs R, Wheatley W, Uribe JW, et al. Intra-articular anterior cruciate ligament reconstruction using patellar tendon allograft in the skeletally immature patient. Arthroscopy 2002;18:824–8.
37. Gaulrapp HM, Haus J. Intraarticular stabilization after anterior cruciate ligament tear in children and adolescents: results 6 years after surgery. Knee Surg Sports Traumatol Arthrosc 2006;14:417–24.
38. Aronowitz ER, Ganley TJ, Goode JR, et al. Anterior cruciate ligament reconstruction in adolescents with open physes. Am J Sports Med 2000;28:168–75.
39. Paletta GA Jr. Special considerations. Anterior cruciate ligament reconstruction in the skeletally immature. Orthop Clin North Am 2003;34:65–77.
40. McCarroll JR, Shelbourne KD, Porter DA, et al. Patellar tendon graft reconstruction for midsubstance anterior cruciate ligament rupture in junior high school athletes. An algorithm for management. Am J Sports Med 1994;22:478–84.
41. Guzzanti V, Falciglia F, Stanitski CL. Physeal-sparing intraarticular anterior cruciate ligament reconstruction in preadolescents. Am J Sports Med 2003;31:949–53.
42. Mohtadi N, Grant J. Managing anterior cruciate ligament deficiency in the skeletally immature individual: a systematic review of the literature. Clin J Sport Med 2006;16: 457–64.
43. Kocher MS, Garg S, Micheli LJ. Physeal sparing reconstruction of the anterior cruciate ligament in skeletally immature prepubescent children and adolescents. J Bone Joint Surg Am 2005;87:2371–9.
44. Kocher MS, Garg S, Micheli LJ. Physeal sparing reconstruction of the anterior cruciate ligament in skeletally immature prepubescent children and adolescents. Surgical technique. J Bone Joint Surg Am 2006;88(Suppl 1; Pt 2):283–93.

Complete Transphyseal Reconstruction of the Anterior Cruciate Ligament in the Skeletally Immature

George A. Paletta Jr, MD

KEYWORDS

- Transphyseal • Anterior Cruciate Ligament • Reconstruction
- Deformities • Immature • Complete

It is now widely accepted that anterior cruciate ligament (ACL) injuries occur in the skeletally immature and that such injuries are increasingly common. While the exact incidence and prevalence are unknown, it is generally accepted that the frequency of such injuries is increasing. Whether this reflects a true increased incidence as a result of increased levels of performance and intensive training by immature athletes or simply an increased recognition of the injury remains unclear. However, factors that are clear regarding ACL injuries in the skeletally immature include the poor prognosis of nonoperative treatment,[1–5] the risk of additional injury in the untreated individual,[3–5] the effects of those additional injuries on the long-term health of the individual's knee, and the unique challenges of surgical treatment in this select group of athletes. Past surgical approaches to the care of the immature athlete with an ACL tear emphasized physeal preservation through nonanatomic reconstructions. Unfortunately, time has proved these techniques to be suboptimal in restoring knee stability and returning an athlete to a level of function that approaches his or her preinjury status. More recent approaches include more anatomic, intra-articular reconstructions including partial physeal sparing and all-epiphyseal techniques that seek to minimize or eliminate risk of injury to the physes and the potential for subsequent angular deformity or leg length discrepancy. Complete transphyseal techniques have been used with good results in the adolescent population but caution and concern have limited the use of such techniques in the prepubescent ACL-injured athlete. The author reviews the current state of the art of transphyseal reconstruction of the ACL in the skeletally immature athlete. The review will include a discussion of the basic science that offers some support for transphyseal reconstruction, past clinical experiences with transphyseal reconstruction in the adolescent population, and current experiences using such

The author has nothing to disclose.
The Orthopedic Center of St. Louis, 14825 North Outer Forty Road, Suite 200, Chesterfield, MO 63017, USA
E-mail address: gpaletta@toc-stl.com

techniques in the preadolescent individual including a focus on exact technical recommendations and clinical outcomes.

BASIC SCIENCE: TRANSPHYSEAL DRILLING, GRAFT TENSIONING, AND RISK OF PHYSEAL INJURY

Of the many unique challenges presented by the surgical treatment of a skeletally immature ACL-injured athlete, none is more daunting than the potential risk of physeal injury. However, both past and more recent basic science investigations offer some evidence to support use of specific techniques to minimize risk of physeal injury when using transphyseal drilling.[6–10] More than 50 years ago, Campbell and colleagues[6] demonstrated that single large drill holes placed across the canine physis and then spanned by cortical bone graft resulted in near complete growth arrest and maximum growth disturbance. However, physeal drill holes of the same diameter that were not bridged by cortical bone graft resulted in minor growth disturbance. In 1994, Guzzanti and colleagues,[7] using a lapine model, investigated the effects of intra-articular ACL reconstruction on physeal growth. The study used a semitendinosus tendon placed through 2-mm tibial and femoral drill holes in skeletally immature rabbits. A tibial drill hole of 2 mm involved 12% of the frontal plane or 4% of the cross-sectional area of the tibial physis. One of the specimens developed tibial epiphysiodesis. A 2-mm femoral drill hole involved 11% of the frontal plane or 3% of the cross-sectional area of the tibial physis. None of the rabbits developed femoral epiphysiodesis. The authors suggested that drill holes that did not exceed these extents of involvement of the tibial and femoral physes had low risk for physeal injury. Stadelmaier and colleagues[8] investigated the effects of a soft tissue graft placed across a physeal drill hole on the risk of physeal arrest and growth disturbance in a dog. In their model, transphyseal drills holes were created and either left empty or filled with a traversing fascia lata graft. Animals were killed at 2 and 16 weeks after the experimental surgical treatment. In those animals whose physes were left nongrafted, 100% developed bone bridges with premature physeal closure and growth disturbance. In those animals grafted with fascia lata, there were no bone bridges, 0% premature physeal closure, and no limb length abnormalities.

Another proposed potential mechanism for physeal injury and growth disturbance following transphyseal ACL reconstruction in the skeletally immature is thought to be related to graft tensioning. Several studies have suggested that graft tensioning across the physis may result in either angular deformity or leg length discrepancy.[9,10] Edwards and colleagues[9] used a canine model to examine the effects of tensioning of an iliotibial band (ITB) transphyseal graft on limb growth. In their model, transphyseal drill holes were spanned using an ITB graft tensioned at 80 Newtons. While no osseous bars or premature physeal closure resulted, the animals developed distal femoral valgus and proximal tibial varus deformities. Unfortunately, the graft tension used in this model is extremely high and probably excessive as it is not representative of the tension typically applied to an ACL graft in the clinical setting. Similar findings were noted in a rabbit model study by Houle and colleagues.[10] However, that study also used a high tension construct that was not thought to be representative of the tension applied in the typical clinical setting. No study examining the effects of more clinically applicable tension levels has been published. In that these studies do not accurately reflect the tension used in the typical clinical setting, it is difficult to extrapolate the results to a risk of growth disturbance in the skeletally immature individual undergoing ACL reconstruction.

A detailed investigation of the femoral origin of the ACL and its relationship to the distal femoral physis was published by Behr and colleagues.[11] This study sought to define the anatomic relationship of the femoral attachment of the ACL to the distal femoral physeal plate in the skeletally immature knee. The study used 12 fresh frozen fetal specimens with gestational age of 23 to 36 weeks and 13 skeletally immature knee specimens with age ranging from 5 to 15 years. The specimens were sectioned in sagittal plane through ACL and physis. The distance from the epiphyseal side of proliferative zone of the physis to the top of the femoral attachment of the ACL was determined and averaged 2.66 ± 0.18 mm (range, 2.34–2.94 mm). In addition, the study demonstrated that this distance remains constant throughout growth. Further-more, the "over-the-top position" is at the same level as the growth plate, suggesting an over-the-top reconstruction would put the physis at risk. The 2.5-mm distance of the proximal portion of the origin of the ACL from the distal femoral physis also suggests that true anatomic reconstruction using a transverse epiphyseal femoral tunnel leaves little room for error without risk for injury to a large area of the physis.

PARTIAL TRANSPHSEAL VERSUS COMPLETE TRANSPHYSEAL RECONSTRUCTION

Many techniques using partial transphyseal drilling have been reported.[12–14] Such techniques are typically hybrid techniques that involve drilling of the tibial physis with avoidance of violation of the femoral physis. Alternatives for femoral placement of the graft include the over-the-top position of transverse epiphyseal drilling distal to the femoral physis. In addition, modifications of the tibial drilling technique include smaller drill holes and more vertically and centrally placed tunnels. These so-called physeal-respecting techniques include reports from Lipscomb and Anderson.[12] Parker and colleagues,[13] and Andrews and colleagues.[14] All series have reported good clinical outcomes, but the series from Parker and colleagues[13] included the report of a 2-cm leg length discrepancy resulting from placement of staples across the physes.

Only one study has reported on a comparison of transphyseal and partial transphyseal reconstruction. Paletta and colleagues[15] reported on a retrospective review of 21 Tanner stage I and II skeletally immature patients undergoing either transphyseal reconstruction (**Fig. 1**) or partial transphyseal reconstruction with a semitendinosus and gracilis autograft. The partial transphyseal group underwent trans-physeal tibial drilling and nonanatomic femoral placement of the graft in the over-the-top position (**Fig. 2A–D**). Fixation in both groups was proximal to the femoral physis and distal to the tibial physis. Patients were followed for a minimum of 24 months. The mean limb growth was 5.9 cm in the over-the-top group and 6.4 cm in the transphyseal group. The over-the-top group had a mean postoperative Lysholm score of 88 versus 96 for the transphyseal group. While there was no leg length discrepancy, angular deformity, or premature physeal closure in either group, there was a significant difference in the stability outcomes of the 2 procedures. In the over-the-top group, 7 of 10 had a positive pivot shift and a mean KT-1000 side-to-side difference of 3.6 mm, with only 1 of 10 having a value of less than 3 mm. In the transphyseal group, only 1 of 11 had a positive pivot shift. The mean KT-1000 side-to-side difference was 1.2 mm, with 0 of 10 having a value of greater than 3 mm. This study suggests that partial transphyseal reconstruction using over-the-top femoral place-ment of the graft does not result in stability equivalent to that of a complete transphyseal reconstruction.

EARLY EXPERIENCES WITH TRANSPHYSEAL RECONSTRUCTIONS

The results of complete transphyseal reconstruction techniques used in skeletally immature athletes have been reported in a number of series.[16–22] In one of the earliest

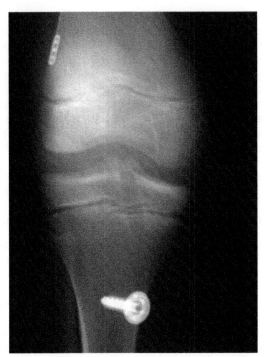

Fig. 1. All transphyseal reconstruction with suspensory femoral fixation and screw and washer tibial fixation.

series, McCarroll and colleagues[16,17] reported on 20 skeletally immature adolescent patients. The patients in this group were of Tanner stage III, IV, and V and not prepubescent individuals. All patients underwent complete transphyseal reconstruction using a patella tendon autograft. McCarroll and colleagues reported 100% of the patients to have stable knees with 90% returning to sports. There were no reported leg length or angular deformities. Matava and Siegel[18] reported on 8 skeletally immature patients undergoing transphyseal reconstruction with hamstring autografts. Again, the study group was composed of mainly adolescent individuals with no physiologic age documentation. The authors reported 8 of 8 returned to sport activities. Three of the 8 had a KT-1000 side-to-side difference of greater than 3 mm. There were no reported physeal arrests or leg length discrepancies. In 2000, Arnowitz[19] reported a series of 19 patients undergoing transphyseal reconstruction using an Achilles allograft. All patients had a bone age of less than 14 years. The mean Lysholm score was 97; 84% returned to sports; and the average KT-1000 side-to-side difference was 1.7 mm. Arnowitz reported no leg length or angular deformities. Fuchs and colleagues[20] reported on 10 patients who underwent transphyseal ACL reconstruction using a patella tendon allograft. The graft included bone plugs. Fixation of the bone plugs was achieved with interference screws placed proximal to the femoral physis and distal to the tibial physis. Patients were followed for 40 months. No growth disturbances were reported. In 2002, Aichroth and colleagues[21] reported on 47 transphyseal reconstructions in 45 patients. Their technique included use of a hamstring autograft with fixation proximal to the femoral physis and distal to the tibial physis. They reported no leg length discrepancies or angular deformities;

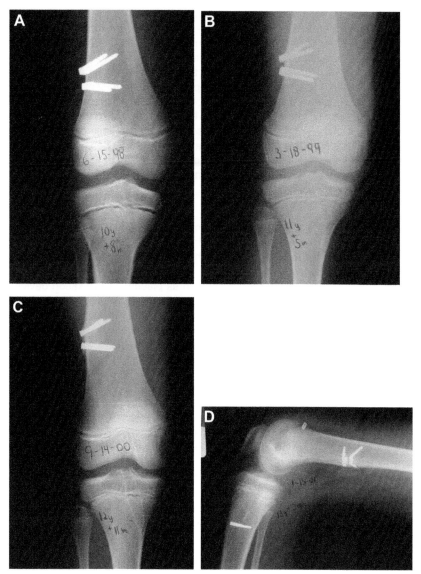

Fig. 2. (*A–D*) Partial transphyseal ACL reconstruction using trans-tibial tunnel and over-the-top femoral graft placement with staple fixation proximal to the physis. Note growth of limb over 27 months as evidenced by migration of staples. Physes remain open and normal in appearance. Lateral view is following revision to complete transphyseal reconstruction due to continued functional instability.

however, their cohort included mainly adolescent patients without documentation of physiologic age (Tanner staging). Most recently, Kocher and colleagues[22] reported on a series of 59 knees in Tanner stage III patients with an average age of 14.7 years. This clearly represents a pubescent or adolescent group of individuals. Reconstruction was performed using a quadruple hamstring autograft with metaphyseal fixation. At a mean follow-up of 3.6 years, the mean International Knee Documentation Committee (IKDC) subjective score was 89.5, and the mean Lysholm score was 91.2. The Lachman test was normal in 51 and nearly normal in 8. The Pivot Shift test was normal in 56 and nearly normal in 3. Kocher and colleagues reported no angular deformities or leg length discrepancies and concluded that transphyseal reconstruction using their technique was a safe procedure in the pubescent adolescent.

These published series suggest that complete transphyseal reconstruction of the ACL is safe in skeletally immature individuals. However, the applicability of these early reports to the skeletally immature prepubescent patient is limited due to multiple shortcomings, including the retrospective nature of some series, series with small numbers of patients, lack of specificity of diagnosis and concomitant pathology, and lack of skeletal or physiologic maturity documentation.

WHERE ARE THE DEFORMITIES?

The most commonly cited reason for avoiding a transphyseal reconstruction in the skeletally immature individual is the risk of physeal damage with resulting leg length discrepancy or angular deformity. While such a risk is clearly possible, there is little documentation of such resulting deformities, and of those that have been reported, most can be attributed to technical errors such as placement of fixation devices or bone plugs across the physis. In the most widely quoted study of deformity after ACL reconstruction in the skeletally immature, Kocher and colleagues[23] reported the results of a survey study of the members of the Herodicus Society. The study reported 15 deformities related to ACL reconstruction yet no denominator was reported; thus, a true incidence could not be determined. More important, technical errors likely accounting for the physeal injury were identifiable in 14 of the 15 cases. There were 8 reported cases of distal femoral valgus with formation of a physeal bar. Three cases had screws across the physis, 3 cases had bone plugs across the physis, and 1 case had a 12-mm tunnel drilled across the physis. The 1 case without an identifiable technical error did not include transphyseal drilling of the femur. In that case, the graft was placed in the over-the-top femoral position. There were 2 reported cases of genu valgum resulting from lateral extra-articular tenodeses with likely tethering of the physis. There were 2 cases of leg length discrepancy with 1 case demonstrating a bone block placed across the physis. The other case was a case of 3 cm of overgrowth of the operative limb. There were also 3 cases of recurvatum with formation of an apophyseal bar. In all 3 cases, there was hardware placed across the tibial tubercle apophysis.

SURGICAL TECHNIQUE OF ANATOMIC, COMPLETE TRANSPHYSEAL ACL RECONSTRUCTION

Based on the basic science data cited earlier and a careful analysis of the limited reports of the clinical outcomes of transphyseal reconstruction of the ACL in skeletally immature patient, the author has been performing complete transphyseal reconstruction of the ACL in prepubescent athletes using a carefully developed technique to minimize violation of the physis and maximize protection against premature physeal arrest. This technique is currently used in all skeletally immature patients who are ultimately indicated for surgical reconstruction regardless of their physiologic or skeletal maturity.

Surgical reconstruction is indicated for any patient who demonstrates associated meniscal pathology at the time of initial presentation or any patient with clear functional instability as indicated by repeated episodes of giving way. Standard diagnostic arthroscopy is performed and concomitant pathology is appropriately addressed. All reasonable attempts should be made to preserve the menisci if the tear pattern is amenable to repair.

Autologous semitendinosus and gracilis hamstrings are used as the graft of choice. Central third patella tendon autograft should be avoided as the use of bone plugs across the physis will induce physeal closure and injury to the anterior tibial tubercle apophysis as a result of harvest may cause a recurvatum deformity. Allograft tissue is also not recommended for use in this population due to the remote risk of disease transmission and evidence of increased rate of failure when used in young, athletic individuals. The hamstring graft is harvested through an anteromedial incision over the pes anserinus at the proximal aspect of the tibial metaphysis. Both the semitendinosus and gracilis are harvested as free tissue grafts and the ends are prepared with No. 2 nonabsorbable suture. Each tendon will be doubled to create a quadruple strand graft. The graft is then sized using sizing cannulas that are of 0.5-mm increments. The smallest cannula that allows passage of the quadruple graft is selected as the drill size. The use of 0.5-mm increment drills is critical to ensure creation of the smallest drill possible to allow passage of the graft. Tight fill of the tunnels with the soft tissue graft is preferable.

A soft tissue notchplasty is performed with care taken to identify the anatomic origin and insertion or femoral and tibial footprints of the ACL. The over-the-top position is not violated and no bone is resected as part of the notchplasty. The tibial guide is placed so that the tunnel aperture will be within the middle of the tibial footprint. The guide is set at as steep an angle as possible in an effort to create a relatively long and vertical tibial tunnel whose origin is far distal to the tibial physis. This allows for the creation of a tibial drill hole that is as close to circular as possible as it crosses the physis. This minimizes the cross-sectional or frontal area of involvement. Drilling is done using a low-speed, high-torque drill. This combination minimizes the risk of heat during drilling and the associated risk of heat necrosis to the physis. Drills and reamers should be passed only once. The femoral tunnel is drilled in a similar manner, again using the smallest acorn-type reamer possible to allow graft passage. The aperture of the femoral tunnel is placed within the footprint of the ACL origin to ensure anatomic reconstruction. A transtibial or anteromedial approach may be used. Care is taken to create as vertical a tunnel as possible with the starting point of the tunnel being within the footprint of the ACL. The creation of a very oblique femoral tunnel should be avoided as this will increase the area of violation of the physis. As on the tibial side, drilling should be done using low speed and high torque. The femoral tunnel should be drilled as long as possible and should extend to but not through the lateral femoral cortex. The femoral cortex is drilled using a smaller drill (typically 4.5 mm) that accompanies the suspensory fixation device of choice that will be used for femoral fixation. Intraoperative fluoroscopy is helpful in confirming placement and position of the drill holes relative to the physes.

The quadruple graft is passed under direct arthroscopic visualization. The maximum length of graft possible (a minimum of 25 mm) should be placed into the femoral tunnel, thereby ensuring that a soft tissue graft is traversing the physis and filling the tunnel. Suspension femoral fixation is used. No fixation device is placed across the femoral physis. Use of cross-fixation devices, interference screws, or expansile devices creating aperture fixation should be avoided. The graft is tensioned in the usual fashion with the knee at about 15 to 20 degrees of flexion. Tibial fixation is achieved distal to the physis. If a long tunnel has been created and there is substantial tunnel length below the proximal tibial physis, an interference screw may be used; however, one must be certain the screw remains below the physis. In most cases, tibial fixation will be achieved using either a ligament staple or by tying the sutures to a screw and post.

Postoperative rehabilitation is identical to that used in skeletally mature patients undergoing ACL reconstruction with the exception of a more prolonged period of postoperative brace immobilization. The rehabilitation program incorporates concepts of progressive physiologic stress on the graft by allowing early motion, weight bearing, and muscle strengthening with care taken to prevent misuse and abuse. Early emphasis is placed on restoring full range of motion and active quadriceps control. Early strengthening includes closed chain kinetic progressive resistive exercises with hamstring and quadriceps co-contraction. Return to functional activities and full sports participation is allowed only when full motion is restored and normal quadriceps-hamstring strength ratios are achieved.

RESULTS OF ANATOMIC TRANSPHYSEAL ACL RECONSTRUCTION IN THE PREPUBESCENT PATIENT

A prospective study of 50 prepubescent, skeletally immature patients undergoing ACL reconstruction using the technique described above has been reported by Paletta and colleagues.[24] The study included 43 boys who were in Tanner Stage I, II, or III and 7 premenarchal girls. The average chronologic age was 11.5 years (range, 7–13 years). All patients underwent reconstruction using quadruple hamstring tendon autograft and following the principles outlined earlier. Follow-up was for a minimum of 3 years and a mean of 4.5 years (range, 3–10). Mean limb growth was 10.4 cm. Twenty-nine of the 50 have been followed to skeletal maturity. The mean postoperative Lysholm score was 94.5, and 47 to 50 were rated normal/nearly normal using the IKDC score. The mean KT-1000 side to side difference was 1.2 mm (range, –2 to 4 mm) with only 3 of 50 having values greater than 3 mm. The pivot shift was negative in 48 of 50, and 49 of 50 reported no functional instability. Return to preinjury level of sports participation was achieved in 44 of 50. Annual full-length standing hip to ankle anteroposterior views of the lower extremities were obtained to measure leg length and angular alignment. There were no leg length discrepancies and no angular deformities noted.

SUMMARY

Complete transphyseal reconstruction of the anterior cruciate ligament in prepubescent, skeletally immature patients must be done using a soft tissue hamstring autograft that spans or traverses the physes and with attention to the principles of tight tunnel fit, use of 0.5-mm incremental reamers with low speed and high torque, creation of a long, central tibial tunnel, avoidance of oblique femoral tunnels, and fixation proximal to the femoral physis and distal to the tibial physis. Intraoperative fluoroscopy is helpful in ensuring optimal tunnel placement and orientation. Reconstruction using these principles offers predictable outcomes of good stability and a high return to preinjury level of function with low risk for iatrogenic physeal injury.

REFERENCES

1. Pressman AD, Letts RM, Jarvis JG. Anterior cruciate ligament tears in children: an analysis of operative versus nonoperative treatment. J Pediatric Orthop 1997;17: 505–11.
2. Graf BK, Lange RH, Fujisaki CK, et al. Anterior cruciate ligament tears in skeletally immature patients: meniscal pathology at presentation and after attempted conservative treatment. Arthroscopy 1992;8:229–33.

3. Janary PM, Nystrom A, Werner S, et al. Anterior cruciate ligament injuries in skeletally immature patients. J Pediatr Orthop 1996;16:673–7.
4. Millett PH, Willis AA, Warren RF. Associated injuries in pediatric and adolescent anterior cruciate ligament tears: does a delay in treatment increase the risk of meniscal tear? Arthoscopy 2002;18:955–99.
5. Mizuta H, Kubota K, Shiraishi M, et al. The conservative treatment of complete tears of the anterior cruciate ligament in skeletally immature patients. J Bone Joint Surg Br 1995;77:890–4.
6. Campbell CJ, Grisolia A, Zanconato G. The effects produced in the cartilaginous epiphyseal plate of immature dogs by experimental surgical trauma. J Bone Joint Surg 1959;41-A:1221–42.
7. Guzzanti V, Falciglia F, Gigante A, et al. The effect of intra-articular ACL reconstruction on the growth plates of rabbits. J Bone Joint Surg Br 1994;76:960–3.
8. Stadelmaler DN, Arnoczky SP, Dodds J, et al. The effect of drilling an ssoft tissue grafting across open growth plates. A histologic study An J Sports Med 1995;23: 431–5.
9. Edwards TB, Greene CC, Baratta RV, et al. The effect of placing a tensioned graft across open growh plates. A gross and histologic analysis. J Bone Joint Surg Am 2001;83:725–34.
10. Houle JB, Letts M, Yang J. Effects of a tensioned tendon graft in a bone tunnel across the rabbit physis. Clin Orhop Relat Res 2001;391:275–81.
11. Behr CT, Potter HG, Paletta GA Jr. The relationship of the femoral origin of the anterior cruciate ligament and the distal femoral physeal plate in the skeletally immature knee. An anatomic study. Am J Sports Med 2001;29:781–7.
12. Lipscomb AB, Anderson AF. Tears of the anterior cruciate ligament in adolescents. J Bone Joint Surg Am 1986;68:19–28.
13. Parker AW, Drez D, Cooper JL. Anterior cruciate ligament injuries in patients with open physes. Am J Sports Med 1994;22:44–7.
14. Andrews M, Noyes FR, Barber-Westin SK. Anterior cruciate ligament allograft reconstruction in the skeletally immature athlete. Am J Sports Med 1994;22:48–54.
15. Paletta GA Jr. Comparison of trans-physeal vs over-the-top reconstruction: is there a difference? Presented at the ACL Study Group. Big Sky, MT, 2005.
16. McCarroll JR, Rettig AC, Shelbourne KD. Anterior cruciate ligament injuries in the young athlete with open physes. Am J Sports Med 1988;16:44–7.
17. McCarroll, JR, Shelbourne KD, Porter DA, et al. Patellar tendon graft reconstruction for midsubstance anterior cruciate ligament rupture in junior high athletes. An algorithm for management. Am J Sports Med 1994;22:478–84.
18. Matava MJ, Siegel MG. Arthoscopic reconstruction of the ACL with semitendinosis-gracilis autograft in skeletally immature adolescent patients. Am J Knee Surg 1997; 10:60–9.
19. Aronowitz ER, Ganley TJ, Goode JR, et al. Anterior cruciate ligament reconstruction in adolescents with open physes. Am J Sports Med 2000;28:168–75.
20. Fuchs R, Wheatley W, Uribe JW, et al. Intra-articular anterior cruciate ligament reconstruction using patellar tendon allograft in the skeletally immature patient. Arthoscopy 2002;18:824–8.
21. Aichroth PM, Patel DV, Zorrilla P. The natural history and treatment of rupture of the anterior cruciate ligament in children and adolescents. A prospective review. J Bone Joint Surg Br 2002;84:38–41.
22. Kocher MS, Smith JT, Zoric BJ, et al. Transphyseal anterior cruciate ligament reconstruction in skeletally immature pubescent adolescents. J Bone Joint Surg Am 2007;89:2632–9.

23. Kocher MS, Saxon HS, Hovis WD, et al. Management and complications of anterior cruciate ligament injuries in skeletally immature patients: survey of the Herodicus Society and The ACL Study Group. J Pediatr Orthop 2002;22:452–7.
24. Paletta GA Jr. Transphyseal ACL reconstruction in the skeletally immature: a prospective study of fifty patients. Presented at the International Pediatric Orthopedic Society Meeting. Orlando, FL, 2009.

Anterior Cruciate Ligament Reconstruction Timing in Children with Open Growth Plates: New Surgical Techniques Including All-Epiphyseal

Eric J. Wall, MD[a],*, Gregory D. Myer, PhD, CSCS[b,c,d,e],
Megan M. May, MD[f]

KEYWORDS

- ACL • Anterior cruciate ligament • Surgery • All-epiphyseal
- Growth plates • Children

INCIDENCE OF ANTERIOR CRUCIATE LIGAMENT TEARS IN YOUNG PATIENTS

Over the past decade, there has been a dramatic increase in the total number of participants in organized youth sports,[1] with up to 63% of sports-related injuries in children aged 6 to 12 years reported as joint sprains, and the majority of these sprains occurring at the knee.[2] Tears of the anterior cruciate ligament (ACL) in young patients are becoming increasingly more recognized.[3–5] In a prospective study of all children with traumatic knee effusions presenting to a pediatric hospital

This study was completed in its entirety at Cincinnati Children's Hospital Medical Center. Research was supported by the Division of Pediatric Orthopaedic Surgery at Cincinnati Children's Hospital Medical Center. No other funding was provided for this study.

The authors have nothing to disclose.

[a] Division of Orthopaedic Surgery, Cincinnati Children's Hospital Medical Center, 3333 Burnet Avenue, Cincinnati, OH 45229-3039, USA

[b] Division of Sports Medicine, Cincinnati Children's Hospital Medical Center, 3333 Burnet Avenue, Cincinnati, OH 45229, USA

[c] Department of Pediatrics and Orthopaedic Surgery, College of Medicine, University of Cincinnati, Cincinnati, OH 45221, USA

[d] Departments of Physiology and Cell Biology, Orthopaedic Surgery, Family Medicine and Biomedical Engineering, The Ohio State University Sports Health & Performance Institute, The Ohio State University, Columbus, OH 43221, USA

[e] Departments of Athletic Training, Sports Orthopaedics, and Pediatric Science, Rocky Mountain University of Health Professions, Provo, UT 84606, USA

[f] Division of Sports Medicine, The Ohio State University, Columbus, OH 43210, USA

* Corresponding author.

E-mail address: Eric.Wall@cchmc.org

Clin Sports Med 30 (2011) 789–800
doi:10.1016/j.csm.2011.07.002
0278-5919/11/$ – see front matter © 2011 Published by Elsevier Inc.

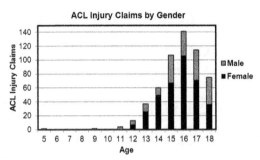

Fig. 1. Chart showing incidence of anterior cruciate ligament tears in data from one insurance company that specifically insures young soccer players. (*Adapted from* Shea KG, Pfeiffer R, Wang JH, et al. Anterior cruciate ligament injury in pediatric and adolescent soccer players: an analysis of insurance data. J Pediatr Orthop 2004;24:623–8; with permission.)

emergency department, 29% of injuries were to the ACL and only 2% were to the tibial eminence.[6] In a consecutive series of children with open growth plates and ACL-type injuries identified on magnetic resonance imaging (MRI), 74% had ACL tears (complete or partial) and 26% had tibial spine fractures.[7] The older children with closing or closed growth plates had a 96% incidence of ACL mid-substance injury and only a 4% incidence of tibial spine fracture.[7] The increased recognition of mid-substance tears in children is probably due to the increased availability and accuracy of pediatric MRI and the increased participation of children in sports, especially basketball, soccer, and football. Mid-substance tears in children younger than 14 years comprise about 1% to 3% of all ACL tears.[8-10] Shea and colleagues[11] reviewed the records of an insurance company specializing in soccer coverage and found that only 2 of 553 ACL tears occurred in children aged 5 to 10 (**Fig. 1**).[11] ACL claims increased rapidly after age 10. These data illustrate that ACL tears are still rare in the very youngest children.

ASSESSING SKELETAL MATURITY

It is critically important to assess skeletal maturity in young athletes who tear their ACL. Because the likelihood of sustaining an ACL injury rises rapidly at skeletal maturity, many young athletes who tear their ACL may be "early bloomers," with bone ages that are far older than their chronologic ages. Researchers find that most ACL tears in skeletally immature patients occur within 6 to 12 months of skeletal maturity.[12]

While chronologic age has been used historically for initial consideration and decision making in the treatment of ACL tears in children and adolescents, it is clear that maturity-related differences in bone development are evident between children of similar ages.[13] The most accurate method of maturity assessment is Tanner staging by a clinician who is skilled and trained in the assessment of secondary sexual characteristics.[14] A hand bone age is a reliable marker if the assessment is focused on the digits rather than on the wrists.[14] The most widely used method of measuring skeletal maturity is through use of the atlas of Greulich and Pyle to match a hand radiograph, but the Tanner-Whitehouse method (TW3), which focuses on the growth plates in the fingers, may be the most reliable method.[14] Bone age is preferred over Tanner staging in the orthopaedic office due to the immediate availability of the radiograph. This avoids social stigma and the questionable reliability of an orthopae-dist performing Tanner staging, which involves careful examination of pubic hair, breast size and shape, or testicular volume. Less reliable methods of maturity assessment are the Risser sign staging of the iliac crest apophysis or the age of menarche.[14] Prior orthopedic studies on ACL reconstruction on children have assessed parental height, secondary sexual characteristics,[15] recent change in foot size,[8] Risser sign, presence of nonpigmented axillary hair,[16] menarchal status,[16] having "wide open" physes, and knee radiographic determination of bone age. The reliability and validity of these methods are not known. Elbow bone age and a simplified staging system based on finger phalangeal maturity may improve accuracy of determining a child's remaining growth.[17–19] A patient's self-assessment of his or her Tanner stage is also not reliable.[20]

Somatic maturational assessments are traditionally the best way to identify rapid adolescent growth.[21] Individually determined percentage of adult height may also be used as a relatively quick and noninvasive indicator of maturity status.[13] The Khamis-Roche method of estimated adult stature was developed from the Fels Longitudinal Study[22] and uses individual stature, mass, age and mid-parental stature in a regression equation for boys and girls. Peak height velocity (PHV) is the maximum growth rate during the adolescent growth spurt; it occurs at approximately age 12 in girls and age 14 in boys, but there can be wide variation among children.[23,24] Serial height measurements can also be reliable if trained personnel perform this measure-ment with a wall-mounted staidiometer. The orthopaedist can assess the child's growth spurt timing by requesting the child's growth curve from his or her primary care physician. Endocrinologists routinely request growth charts from the primary care referring physician when they see a new patient in consultation.

The following case illustrates the importance of determining skeletal maturity in the clinical decision-making process for a skeletal immature patient with an ACL injury. A 10-year-old girl who tore her ACL was referred for a pediatric ACL reconstruction. She appeared more physically mature than age 10. A left hand bone age radiograph was obtained, which revealed that her skeletal maturity matched that of a 14-year-old girl with the finger growth plates closed (**Fig. 2**A). For comparison, **Fig. 2**B shows a radiograph of another 10-year-old girl with a true bone age of 10 with wide open finger growth plates. The ACL-injured girl with the advanced bone age had knee radio-graphs that showed that her knee growth plates were also closing. Due to her skeletal maturity, as confirmed by a bone age study, she could undergo an adult-style reconstruction through the growth plates with no risk of growth disturbance even at the chronologic age of 10 (see **Figs. 2**C, D). This case illustrates the importance of accurately assessing the skeletal maturity in a child and the dramatic effect it can have on treatment.

NATURAL HISTORY OF NONOPERATIVE TREATMENT OF IMMATURE ANTERIOR CRUCIATE LIGAMENT TEARS

The natural history of children with complete mid-substance ACL tears who return to sports without reconstruction is very poor, with some children showing osteoarthritic changes on radiography in less than 12 years postinjury.[25–29] These children have recurrent instability episodes, meniscal and articular cartilage damage, and poor satisfaction with their sports performance.[25] Studies show that 21% to 100% of pediatric patients who sustain a torn ACL suffer a meniscal tear.[5] A delay in ACL reconstruction appears to increase the incidence of meniscal tears[26,27] and may make an originally repairable meniscus tear, irreparable. The long-term results of ACL-injured patients with meniscal damage is much worse

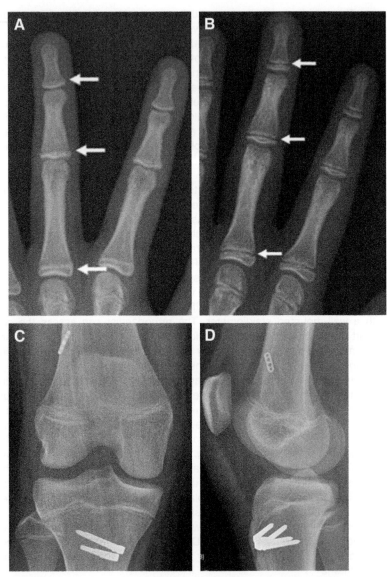

Fig. 2. (*A*) A 10-year-old girl who tore her anterior cruciate ligament (ACL) who has a bone age of 14. Arrows show that finger growth plates are closed or closing. (*B*) Radiograph for comparison of a 10-year-old girl who has a bone age of 10 years. Arrows point to open growth plates of the fingers. (*C*) Anteroposterior radiograph of the 10-year-old girl, who underwent an "adult-style" ACL reconstruction because her bone age was 14 years and she had minimal (0.4 cm) of knee growth remaining (from **Fig. 4**). If she had a 10-year bone age, she would have had 6.7 cm of knee growth remaining (from **Fig. 4**). (*D*) Lateral radiograph of same postoperative knee showing a soft tissue graft that crosses her closing growth plate (transphyseal) but with fixation that does not cross her closing growth plates (*Courtesy of* Eric Wall, MD, Cincinnati, OH).

than for those with intact menisci.[30–32] Poor meniscal condition plus an ACL tear portends osteoarthritis.

In general, children's increased activity levels make them much more reliant on the stability provided by the ACL than adults. Most children in team sports will practice and compete more than 200 hours per year, which far exceeds that of an adult weekend or weeknight warrior who plays on a recreational basketball team once or twice a week. Most ACL-deficient children who try to return to sports without reconstruction have recurrent episodes of instability, which may damage the meniscus and/or joint surface cartilage, ultimately leading to premature knee arthritis. There are 2 types of children who present in clinic with a ruptured ACL: those children who play sports and those who do not. Unfortunately, a high percentage of children who tear their ACL have a strong inborn desire to play high action cutting sports. Persuading this type of athlete to avoid the cutting sports of basketball, soccer, football, wrestling, lacrosse, and volleyball is usually an unrealistic option. It can be nearly impossible for parents and teachers to enforce strict sports abstinence. Bracing and physical therapy cannot prevent reinjury if the child returns to cutting sports. Thus, delaying reconstruction until skeletal maturity is only a valid option if the child strictly avoids cutting sports and does not have recurrent knee instability episodes.[12,33]

OPERATIVE TREATMENT

Surgery-induced growth disturbance of the knee, the fastest growing joint in the body, can occur via 2 methods. It is well known that a bone bridge can form across the growth plate, which can halt all growth and produce a short or crooked leg. Animal models of immature ACL reconstruction rarely show evidence of a bone bridge across the growth plate as long as the tunnel area comprises 7% or less of the total area of the growth plate and the tunnel is filled with a soft tissue graft under minimal tension. Several authors recommend drilling vertical bone tunnels through the growth plate to minimize the cross-sectional area of the growth plate damage.[34–36] Unfortunately, vertical bone tunnels can lead to vertical graft placement, which is nonanatomic, predisposing the athlete to postoperative rotational instability. This can trigger a cascade of giving-way episodes, cartilage damage, and subsequent knee arthritis. Bone blocks from a patellar tendon graft should not cross an open growth plate, nor should a fixation device such as an interference screw (**Fig. 3**A). In the second, lesser-known method of growth disturbance, the graft itself tethers the growth plate against future growth without the formation of a bony bar (see **Fig. 3**B). This occurs in both immature animal models and in children when a securely fixed and tensioned ACL graft is placed across the growth plate of the femur or tibia as in an adult-style reconstruction.[37–41] This mechanism is similar to that used to guide growth with knee staples and screw plates, in which the devices stop growth without actually producing a bone bridge across the growth plate. In animal models, a securely fixed and tensioned soft tissue graft that crosses the growth plate frequently disturbs growth. Conversely, in other animal studies on immature animals with minimal tensioning of the graft, no growth disturbance is evident.[42,43] Unfortunately, techniques that include low tension of a graft in children and adolescents would not restore joint stability and may predispose their knee to recurrent instability episodes. Meller and colleagues[44] showed no growth disturbance with an adult-style soft tissue reconstruction placed through tunnels in the growth plate, but animals had persistent ACL side-to-side laxity of 3.5 mm at 6 months. Several studies on immature animals in which adult-style tunnels cross the growth plate and are filled with a tensioned soft

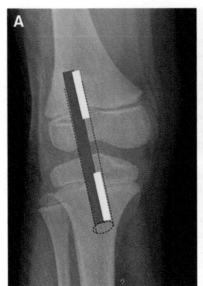 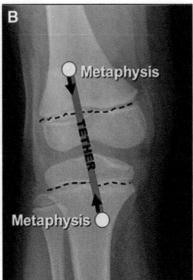

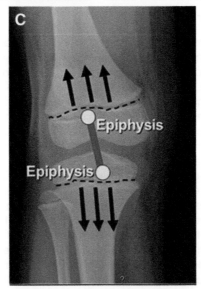

Fig. 3. (A) Immature knee with patella tendon graft in which the bone plugs (represented by the *yellow bars*) span the growth plate. This should be avoided in children with wide open growth plates due to bone plugs causing a bony bar across the growth plate. (B) A solidly fixed and tensioned graft can potentially cause a tether to the growth of the knee, without causing a bony bar to form. White arrows point to the epiphysis. Dashed lines overlie the growth plates. (C) An "all-epiphyseal" anterior cruciate ligament reconstruction places the tunnels, the graft, and the fixation all within the epiphysis in an anatomic fashion. This allows for future growth without the tether effect on the growth plates (*Courtesy of* Eric Wall, MD, Cincinnati, OH).

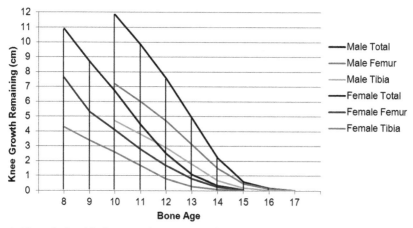

Fig. 4. The relationship between bone age and growth remaining in the knee. Once a girl reaches a bone age of 13, with only 1.1 cm of total knee growth remaining, and a boy reaches a bone age of 14½, with only 1.4 cm of total knee growth remaining, it is usually safe to perform an adult-style anterior cruciate ligament reconstruction with a soft tissue graft. (*Data from* Green WT, Anderson M. Experiences with epiphyseal arrest in correcting discrepancies in length of the lower extremities in infantile paralysis: A method of predicting effect. J Bone Joint Surg Am 1947;29:659–78.)

tissue graft have shown a high graft rupture rate, likely due to the graft failing from the force exerted by growth of the growth plates.[40,41]

The ACL is a collagen-rich cable that links the knee from the epiphysis of the femur to the epiphysis of the tibia. Hence, the native ACL may be described as "all-epiphyseal," a term that recognizes the true pediatric anatomy of the ACL with its origin and insertion only in the epiphysis (see **Fig. 3**C). An "adult-style" transphyseal ACL reconstruction, whether single bundle or double bundle, violates the child's knee anatomy because graft tunnels and fixation devices extend into the metaphyseal regions of the distal femur and proximal tibia. In doing so, the graft spans the child's growth plate. A 10-year-old boy who tears his ACL has almost 12 cm of total growth remaining in his knee (total from the femur and tibia growth plates); (**Fig. 4**). This means that a graft securely fixed into the metaphysis of the femur and tibia must stretch 12 cm from age 10 until age 17. This is physiologically improbable given that the native ACL does not stretch or grow much from birth until maturity. In theory, it is also unlikely that a graft that is securely fixed into the metaphysis would only incorporate into the epiphyseal portion of a transphyseal bone tunnel (exclusively aperture incorporation) and then slide through the physeal and metaphyseal portion of the tunnel to allow growth. Because the failure load of a quadruple adult cadaveric graft is 4090 N,[45] this force will easily tether all femoral and tibial growth before the graft breaks. The force to suppress growth is estimated at 495 N per physis in a child.[46] Metaphyseal fixation is not a problem in adults without a growth plate, but in the child, this carries a small yet serious risk of growth disturbance. In the largest report on ACL growth disturbance in children, 20% of all cases were traced to this "tether effect."[47]

Anderson[48] pioneered a new technique in ACL reconstruction in children and termed it "transepiphyseal." In his technique, the femoral and tibial tunnels are drilled entirely within the epiphysis, avoiding disruption of the growth plate (**Fig. 5**). His

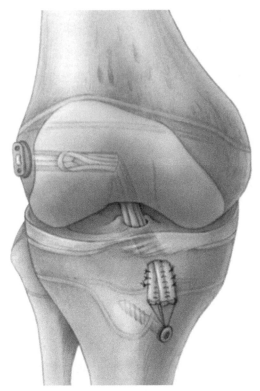

Fig. 5. Transepiphyseal anterior cruciate ligament reconstruction in which the tunnels and the graft are placed within the epiphysis and do not penetrate the growth plate. The tibial graft is fixed to the metaphysic. (*From* Anderson AF. Transepiphyseal replacement of the anterior cruciate ligament using quadruple hamstring grafts in skeletally immature patients. J Bone Joint Surg Am 2004;86:201–9; with permission.)

preliminary report on 12 children showed no clinically relevant growth disturbance despite a 16.5-cm increase in body height. Although Anderson's revolutionary technique relies on post fixation in the tibial metaphysis, it has been modified to eliminate the tibial fixation that spans the growth plate (**Fig. 6**A–D). The graft, the bone tunnels, and fixation can be placed entirely within the epiphysis (all-epiphyseal), which theoretically is the best way to minimize the risk of growth disturbance in an ACL-deficient child. However, even with an "all-epiphyseal" ACL reconstruction, a slight risk of growth disturbance exists due to the proximity of the epiphyseal bone tunnels to the growth plate, which could cause inadvertent damage to the growth plate during drilling. Surgery through the periosteum near a growth plate could also stimulate growth and cause a longer leg. The margin for error when drilling "all-epiphyseal" bone tunnels can be only 1 to 2 mm.[49] An "all-epiphyseal" ACL reconstruction technique places the graft at the native ACL's anatomic attachment points on the femoral and tibial epiphyses. It also allows for immediate postoperative weight bearing, no restriction of motion, and aggressive rehabilitation of the knee similar to adult protocols. Brace wear is not mandatory after "all-epiphyseal" ACL reconstruction, and full return to every sport is permitted after knee rehabilitation.

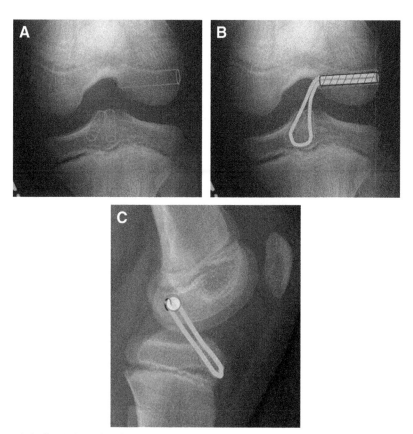

Fig. 6. (*A*) All-epiphyseal technique in which the tunnels are placed in the epiphysis. The tibial tunnel is split into 2 tunnels. This double tunnel gives the advantage of low-profile solid fixation over the intervening cortical bone bridge. It also reduces the tunnel size from 7 to 8 mm to 5 mm, which increases the margin of safety between the growth plate and the joint when drilling the tibial epiphysis. (*B*) While maintaining appropriate tension of the graft, an interference screw is placed from the outside into the femoral tunnel for solid femoral fixation. (*C*) Lateral illustration of an anatomic "all-epiphyseal" graft placement. The looped end of the graft is fixed over the tibial epiphysis bone bridge between the double tunnels, and an interference screw is placed in the femoral tunnel (*Courtesy of* Eric Wall, MD, Cincinnati, OH).

Although the "all-epiphyseal" ACL reconstruction described in this article is a new surgical procedure without long-term outcome data, it holds the theoretical advantage over an adult-style ACL reconstruction in that it does not cross or disrupt the growth plate. For children, treatment decisions for ACL tears should be based on bone age rather than the child's actual chronologic age. Given its theoretical safety benefits and its early clinical success, an "all-epiphyseal ACL" reconstruction may be the safest approach for boys with a bone age less than 14½ and girls with a bone age less than 13 who wish to return to cutting sports. Skeletally immature athletes with bone ages greater than these can safely undergo an adult-style ACL reconstruction with a soft tissue graft as long as the fixation devices do not cross the growth plate.[49] The safest timing of an ACL reconstruction in a young active athlete may be shortly after injury. Anatomic all-epiphyseal techniques minimize the risk of growth disturbance from surgery and minimize the risk of cartilage reinjury from a recurrent unstable knee.

REFERENCES

1. NCYS report on trends and participation in organized youth sports. Available at: http://www.ncys.org/pdfs/2008/2008-ncys-market-research-report.pdf. Accessed December 12, 2010.
2. Gallagher SS, Finison K, Guyer B, et al. The incidence of injuries among 87,000 Massachusetts children and adolescents: results of the 1980–81 Statewide Childhood Injury Prevention Program Surveillance System. Am J Public Health 1984; 74(12):1340–7.
3. Dorizas JA, Stanitski CL. Anterior cruciate ligament injury in the skeletally immature. Orthop Clin N Am 2003;34:355–63.
4. Bales CP, Guettler JH, Moorman CT. Anterior cruciate ligament injuries in children with open physes. Am J Sports Med 2004;32(8):1978–85.
5. Mohtadi N, Grant J. Managing anterior cruciate ligament deficiency in the skeletally immature individual: a systematic review of the literature. Clin J Sport Med 2006;16: 457–64.
6. Luhmann SJ. Acute traumatic knee effusions in children and adolescents. J Pediatr Orthop 2003;23:199–202.
7. Prince JS, Laor T, Bean JA. MRI of anterior cruciate ligament injuries and associated findings in the pediatric knee: changes with skeletal maturation. AJR Am J Roentgenol 2005;185:756–62.
8. Pavlovich R, Goldberg SH, Bach BR. Adolescent ACL injury: treatment considerations. J Knee Surg 2004;17:79–93.
9. DeLee JC, Curtis R. Anterior cruciate ligament insufficiency in children. Clin Orthop Relat Res 1983;172:112–8.
10. Lipscomb AB, Anderson AF. Tears of the anterior cruciate ligament in adolescents. J Bone Joint Surg Am 1986;68:19–28.
11. Shea KG, Pfeiffer R, Wang JH, et al. Anterior cruciate ligament injury in pediatric and adolescent soccer players: an analysis of insurance data. J Pediatr Orthop 2004;24: 623–8.
12. Woods GW, O'Connor DP. Delayed anterior cruciate ligament reconstruction in adolescents with open physes. Am J Sports Med 2004;32(1):201–10.
13. Malina RM, Cumming SP, Morano PJ, et al. Maturity status of youth football players: A noninvasive estimate. Med Sci Sports Exerc 2005;37(6):1044–52.
14. Sanders JO. Maturity indicators in spinal deformity. J Bone Joint Surg Am 2007;89: 14–20.
15. Matava MJ, Siegel MG. Arthroscopic reconstruction of the ACL with semitendinosus-gracilis autograft in skeletally immature adolescent patients. Am J Knee Surg 1997; 10:60–9.
16. Fuchs R, Wheatley W, Uribe JW, et al. Intra-articular anterior cruciate ligament reconstruction using patellar tendon allograft in the skeletally immature patient. Arthroscopy J Arthros Relat Surg 2002;18(8):824–8.
17. Diméglio A, Charles YP, Daures J, et al. Accuracy of the Sauvegrain method in determining skeletal age during puberty. J Bone Joint Surg Am 2005;87:1689–96.
18. Charles YP, Diméglio A, Canavese F, et al. Skeletal age assessment from the olecranon for idiopathic scoliosis at Risser Grade 0. J Bone Joint Surg Am 2007;89:2737–44.

19. Sanders JO, Khoury JG, Kishan S, et al. Predicting scoliosis progression from skeletal maturity: a simplified classification during adolescence. J Bone Joint Surg Am 2008;90:540–53.
20. Desmangles JC, Lappe JM, Lipacqewski G, et al. Accuracy of pubertal Tanner staging self-reporting. J Pediatr Endocrinol Metab 2006;19(3):213–21.
21. Malina RM, Bouchard C. Timing and sequence of changes in growth, maturation, and performance during adolescence. In: Bouchard MA, editor. Growth, maturation, and physical activity. Champaign (IL): Human Kinetics; 1991. p. 267–72.
22. Khamis HJ, Roche AF. Predicting adult stature without using skeletal age: the Khamis-Roche method. Pediatrics 1994;94(4 Pt 1):504–7.
23. Tanner JM, Whitehouse RH, Marubini E, et al. The adolescent growth spurt of boys and girls of the Harpenden growth study. Ann Hum Biol 1976;3(2):109–26.
24. Rowland TW. Exercise and children's health. Champaign (IL): Human Kinetics; 1990.
25. Angel KR, Hall DJ. Anterior cruciate ligament injury in children and adolescents. Arthroscopy J Arthrosc Relat Surg 1989;5(3):197–200.
26. Graf BK, Lange RH, Fujisaki CK, et al. Anterior cruciate ligament tears in skeletally immature patients: meniscal pathology at presentation and after attempted conservative treatment. Arthroscopy J Arthrosc Relat Surg 1992;8(2):229–33.
27. Millett PJ, Willis AA, Warren RF. Associated injuries in pediatric and adolescent anterior cruciate ligament tears: does a delay in treatment increase the risk of meniscal tear? Arthroscopy J Arthrosc Relat Surg 2002;18(9):955–9.
28. Aichroth PM, Patel DV, Zorrilla P. The natural history and treatment of rupture of the anterior cruciate ligament in children and adolescents: a prospective review. J Bone Joint Surg Br 2002;84:38–41.
29. Kannus P, Järvinen M. Knee ligament injuries in adolescents: eight year follow-up of conservative management. J Bone Joint Surg Br 1988;70:772–6.
30. Shelbourne KD, Gray T, Wiley BV. Results of transphyseal anterior cruciate ligament reconstruction using patellar tendon autograft in Tanner Stage 3 or 4 adolescents with clearly open growth plates. Am J Sports Med 2004;32:1218–22.
31. Magnussen RA, Mansour AA, Carey JL, et al. Meniscus status at anterior cruciate ligament reconstruction associated with radiographic signs of osteoarthritis at 5- to 10-year follow-up: a systematic review. J Knee Surg 2009;22(4):347–57.
32. Wu WH, Hackett T, Richmond JC. Effects of meniscal and articular surface status on knee stability, function, and symptoms after anterior cruciate ligament reconstruction: A long-term prospective study. Am J Sports Med 2002;30(6):845–50.
33. Janarv PM, Nyström A, Werner S, et al. Anterior cruciate ligament injuries in skeletally immature patients. J Pediatr Orthop 1996;16(5):673–7.
34. Lo IKY, Kirkley A, Fowler PJ, et al. The outcome of operatively treated anterior cruciate ligament disruptions in the skeletally immature child. Arthroscopy J Arthrosc Relat Surg 1997;13(5):627–34.
35. Kercher J, Xerogeanes J, Tannenbaum A, et al. Anterior cruciate ligament reconstruction in the skeletally immature: an anatomical study utilizing 3-dimensional magnetic resonance imaging reconstructions. J Pediatr Orthop 2009;29:124–9.
36. Kocher MS, Hovis WD, Curtin MJ, et al. Anterior cruciate ligament reconstruction in skeletally immature knees: an anatomical study. Am J Orthop (Belle Mead NJ) 2005;34(6):285–90.
37. Kocher MS, Mandiga R, Klingele K, et al. Anterior cruciate ligament injury versus tibial spine fracture in the skeletally immature knee: a comparison of skeletal maturation and notch width index. J Pediatr Orthop 2004;24:185–8.

38. Edwards TB, Greene CC, Baratta RV, et al. The effect of placing a tensioned graft across open growth plates: a gross and histologic analysis. J Bone Joint Surg Am 2001;83(5):725–34.
39. Houle J, Letts M, Yang J. Effects of a tensioned tendon graft in a bone tunnel across the rabbit physis. Clin Orthop Relat Res 2001;391:275–81.
40. Ono T, Wada Y, Takahashi K, et al. Tibial deformities and failures of anterior cruciate ligament reconstruction in immature rabbits. J Orthop Sci 1998;3:150–5.
41. Chudik SC, Beasley LS, Potter HG, et al. The influence of femoral technique for graft placement on anterior cruciate ligament reconstruction using a skeletally immature canine model with a rapidly growing physis. Arthroscopy J Arthrosc Relat Surg 2007;23(12):1309–19.
42. Stadelmaier DM, Arnoczky SP, Dodds J, et al. The effect of drilling and soft tissue grafting across open growth plates: a histologic study. Am J Sports Med 1995;23(4): 431–5.
43. Meller R, Willbold E, Hesse E, et al. Histologic and biomechanical analysis of anterior cruciate ligament graft to bone healing in skeletally immature sheep. Arthroscopy J Arthrosc Relat Surg 2008;24(11):1221–31.
44. Meller R, Brandes G, Drögemüller C, et al. Graft remodeling during growth following anterior cruciate ligament reconstruction in skeletally immature sheep. Arch Orthop Trauma Surg 2009;129:1037–46.
45. Hamner DL, Brown CH, Steiner ME, et al. Hamstring tendon grafts for reconstruction of the anterior cruciate ligament: biomechanical evaluation of the use of multiple strands and tensioning techniques. J Bone Joint Surg Am 1999;81:549–57.
46. Bylski-Austrow D, Wall EJ, et al. Growth plate forces in the adolescent human knee: a radiographic and mechanical study of epiphyseal staples. J Pediatr Orthop 2001; 21:817–23.
47. Kocher MS, Saxon HS, Hovis WD, et al. Management and complications of anterior cruciate ligament injuries in skeletally immature patients: Survey of the Herodicus Society and the ACL Study Group. J Pediatr Orthop 2002;22:452–7.
48. Anderson AF. Transepiphyseal replacement of the anterior cruciate ligament in skeletally immature patients: a preliminary report. J Bone Joint Surg Am 2003;85: 1255–63.
49. Aronowitz ER, Ganley TJ, Goode JR, et al. Anterior cruciate ligament reconstruction in adolescents with open physes. Am J Sports Med 2000;28:168–75.
50. Anderson AF. Transepiphyseal replacement of the anterior cruciate ligament using quadruple hamstring grafts in skeletally immature patients. J Bone Joint Surg Am 2004;86:201–9.

Anterior Cruciate Ligament Reconstruction in the Young Athlete: A Treatment Algorithm for the Skeletally Immature

Matthew D. Milewski, MD[a], Nicholas A. Beck, BS[b],
J. Todd Lawrence, MD, PhD[b], Theodore J. Ganley, MD[b],*

KEYWORDS

- Anterior cruciate ligament • ACL reconstruction
- Sports medicine • Skeletally immature

Injury to the anterior cruciate ligament (ACL) in the skeletally immature was once considered rare, and it was widely held that tibial spine avulsions rather than ligament ruptures occur in this young population. The incidence of ACL rupture in skeletally immature individuals sustaining a knee injury has historically been reported as 1% to 3.4%.[1-4] In young athletes presenting with hemarthrosis, however, the incidence of ACL rupture has been reported to be between 26% and 65%.[5-9] As imaging and clinical awareness of injuries in young athletes has improved, the diagnosis and reported incidence of ACL injury has increased. The rate of ACL injury in patients with open physes has recently been shown to approach the rate of tibial spine fractures and traumatic ACL disruption has also been described in children as young as 4 years of age.[10,11]

RATIONALE FOR ACL RECONSTRUCTION

Delaying surgical reconstruction until close to skeletal maturity has been the traditionally recommended treatment for ACL injuries in the skeletally immature.[4,12-20] Longer term follow-up, however, has shown an increased risk of meniscal damage, osteochondral damage, chronic instability, and a decreased ability to resume high-level athletics. Chronic instability in the ACL-deficient knee of a skeletally immature

[a] Division of Orthopaedic Surgery, Children's Hospital of Los Angeles, 4650 Sunset Boulevard, MS #69, Los Angeles, CA 90027, USA
[b] Division of Orthopaedic Surgery, The Children's Hospital of Philadelphia, 34th and Civic Center Boulevard, Philadelphia, PA 19104, USA
* Corresponding author.
E-mail address: ganley@email.chop.edu

Clin Sports Med 30 (2011) 801–810
doi:10.1016/j.csm.2011.08.001
0278-5919/11/$ – see front matter © 2011 Elsevier Inc. All rights reserved.

athlete has been shown by multiple investigators to result in an increased risk of meniscal damage.[3,21–24] Graf and colleagues[13] noted that, for young athletes with an ACL-deficient knee, bracing alone does not prevent meniscal tears in the absence of major activity restriction. Suture techniques for primary repair of the ACL have also been shown to be ineffective in preventing continued instability in these patients.[1,21,22]

Delay in operative treatment of the ACL-deficient knee in skeletally immature patients may also have significant repercussions. A recent study from the Children's Hospital of Philadelphia evaluated patients under the age of 14 at the time of ACL reconstruction. In the group with a delay in treatment of longer than 12 weeks to surgery odds ratios from logistic regression analysis revealed that this group was 4 times more likely to have irreparable medial meniscal tears at the time of surgery.[25,26]

POTENTIAL COMPLICATIONS OF ACL RECONSTRUCTION

Concerns over potential complications of ACL reconstruction in the skeletally immature have dissuaded many orthopedic surgeons from operative treatment of these injuries. In skeletally immature patients with wide open physes, the most significant complication of ACL reconstruction is considered to be growth arrest with associated angular deformity and leg-length discrepancy. The distal femoral physis produces approximately 70% of femoral growth, averaging 1.0 cm per year and the proximal tibial physis contributes 60% of tibial growth, averaging 0.9 cm per year.[27]

Multiple studies have examined the risks associated with transphyseal graft placement in animal models. Guzzanti and colleagues[28] placed transphyseal soft tissue grafts and produced valgus deformities and leg-length discrepancy from tibial physeal damage, but noted no femoral deformities. Contrary to the findings in these studies, Stadelmaier and colleagues[29] found no evidence of growth disturbance when a soft tissue graft was placed in the transphyseal drill hole although, these grafts were not tensioned. Edwards and colleagues[28] and Houle and colleagues[30] showed significant deformity with placement of tensioned transphyseal grafts. They concluded that the proximal tibia is most vulnerable to growth arrest, soft-tissue grafts are not protective especially when tensioned, larger tunnels led to increased deformity, and the tunnels should be kept as small as possible (their preference was <1% of the physeal area).

Several authors have reported upon growth disturbances associated with operative treatment of ACL injuries in skeletally immature patients.[3,31,32] In 2002, Kocher and colleagues[31] surveyed members of the Herodicus Society and the ACL Study Group and reported 15 cases of growth disturbances, including 8 valgus deformities from arrest of the lateral distal femoral physis, 3 cases of tibial recurvatum from arrest of the tibial tubercle, 2 cases of genu valgum without frank physeal arrest, and 2 cases of leg-length discrepancy. Risk factors for growth arrest and angular deformity included hardware fixation across the physis, bone plugs across the physis, and lateral extra-articular tenodesis. A recently reported meta-analysis looking at the risk of growth disturbance following ACL reconstruction in patients with open growth plates noted an overall risk of growth disturbance of 1.8% in case series reported in the literature.[33]

Both clinical and basic science studies provide the basis for the current, commonly accepted principles to minimize the risk of growth disturbance with ACL reconstruction in the skeletally immature. Bone plugs and hardware should not cross the physis. Disruption of the perichondrial ring should be avoided and trauma to the tissues surrounding the perichondrial ring should be minimized. Drill holes across the physis should be as small and central in the physis as possible, and caution should be employed when tensioning a soft tissue graft across the physis if there is significant growth remaining.

ASSESSMENT OF SKELETAL MATURITY

An accurate assessment of skeletal maturity is important when considering surgical options for the ACL-deficient knee in young patients, because remaining growth dictates the magnitude of potential complications. Tanner and Whitehouse[34] correlated standards for height, weight, height velocity, and weight velocity with physiologic signs of development. Radiographic methods to assess skeletal maturity include the use of Risser staging of iliac crest ossification and most commonly bone age as determined from hand radiographs.[35] Although Tanner staging is most commonly used by pediatricians, it is not often practical or well-accepted in the orthopedic office setting. Because radiographs are widely available in orthopedic offices, bone age determination using the Greulich and Pyle atlas is most commonly used among orthopedic surgeons. Self-Tanner staging, Tanner staging intraoperatively, and growth relative to family members have also been used as a supplement to bone age by the authors. Further discussion of age in this article refers to bone age based on the Greulich and Pyle atlas.[35]

OPERATIVE TECHNIQUES

Once the decision for operative management of the ACL-deficient knee in the skeletally immature patient has been made, the surgeon must decide on the optimal surgical procedure for the patient and their family. In addition to traditional techniques for ACL reconstruction, there are several unique techniques that are growth plate respecting.

Physeal-sparing techniques were initially described by DeLee and Curtis[2] using patellar tendon grafts without drill holes and by Brief,[36] and Parker and colleagues[37] using hamstring tendon grafts. Guzzanti and colleagues[38] and Anderson[39] have also described physeal sparing hamstring tendon graft fixation techniques. Anderson's technique incorporates a quadrupled hamstring graft tensioned across epiphyseal tunnels in the distal femur and proximal tibia. Femoral fixation was achieved with a cortical button and tibial fixation was achieved with a screw and post construct. Both of these techniques require extra-osseous tensioning of the graft across the tibial physis.

More recently, the authors of this manuscript have described an all-epiphyseal ACL reconstruction technique[40] (**Fig. 1**). This procedure utilizes direct imaging and 3-dimensional analysis of the femoral guide wire and tibial tunnels relative to the femoral and tibial physes to minimize injury risk. A limited-cut, low-dose, intraoperative computed tomography (O-arm; Medtronic, Inc, Minneapolis, MN, USA) is used to create images for the three dimensional analysis (**Fig. 2**). The femoral tunnel is drilled and the graft is secured using a standard cannulated reamer over a pin and interference screw over a guide wire. Tibial tunnel creation and fixation is performed with a drill followed by an interference screw both of which are placed in a retrograde manner (RetroScrew, Arthrex Inc, Naples, FL, USA).

A physeal-sparing combined intra-articular and extra-articular reconstruction with autogenous iliotibial band was developed and reported on in short- and long-term series by Kocher and colleagues[41] in prepubescent children, staged Tanner 1 or 2 (average age 10.3 chronological age). This reconstruction technique has an intra-articular portion as well as a lateral extra-articular iliotibial band reconstruction to help functionally control rotation as originally described by Losee and colleagues.[42] It does avoid physeal tunnels, which is an important consideration in the youngest patients with ACL tears requiring reconstruction.

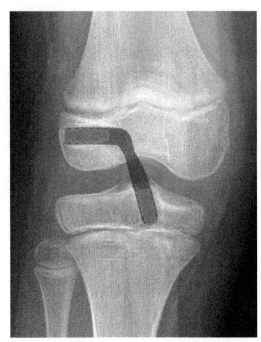

Fig. 1. The Ganley/Lawrence all-epiphyseal ACL reconstruction with tunnel placement, with fixation within the epiphyses.

In addition to these uniquely physeal-sparing techniques, ACL reconstruction with subtle variations to traditional transphyseal techniques have been advocated in skeletally immature patients who are approaching skeletal maturity where the potential for growth disturbance is lower.[24,43,44] Both the Boston and Philadelphia

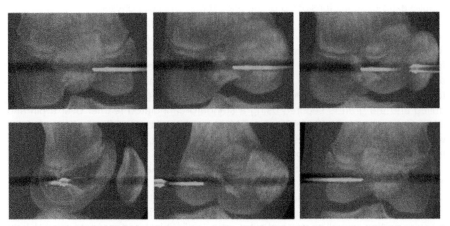

Fig. 2. Intraoperative, 3-dimensional computed tomography allows excellent visualization of the femoral and tibial tunnel placement relative to the physes. Three-dimensional computed tomography reconstruction shows the guide pin in the distal femoral epiphysis; the image is rotated from left to right.

groups have also shown that transphyseal hamstring autograft ACL reconstruction in Tanner stage 3 adolescents resulted in no angular deformities or leg-length discrepancies.[24,45] Ganley and colleagues have shown similar results with transphyseal techniques for ACL reconstruction in adolescent patients relative to the results reported in adult patients.[43] In addition, they have shown that concomitant medial collateral ligament injury with ACL injury in the skeletally immature athlete can be treated with ACL reconstruction and medial collateral ligament bracing as in adult patients.[44]

An important consideration when evaluating the safety of the transphyseal technique for skeletally immature ACL reconstruction is that most series reported in the literature generally used transtibial drilling techniques with very vertical, femoral tunnels. Although ACL reconstructions with a vertically placed femoral graft can provide a subjective sense of knee stability and allow for a high level of return to sports, recent data have revealed that a vertical graft position is typically outside the native ACL footprint and thus does not fully restore the normal biomechanics of the knee as well as a graft positioned more in the center of the anatomic ACL footprint (**Fig. 3**A).[46,47] Placing the graft in the center of the anatomic femoral footprint is most easily accomplished utilizing independent femoral drilling techniques via accessory medial

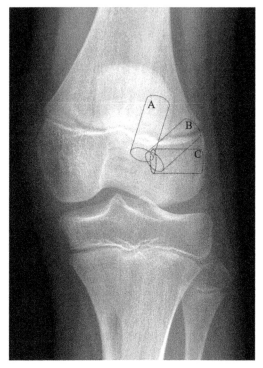

Fig. 3. The amount and location of femoral physis effected using different operative techniques. (*A*) The location of a vertically orientated tunnel, which affects less of the femoral physis but is typically outside of the native ACL footprint. (*B*) The location of a classic anatomic accessory medial portal, or outside in technique, that places the tunnel anatomically in the ACL footprint but affects a large portion of the distal femoral physis. (*C*) The location of a femoral tunnel, which is in the anatomic center of the ACL footprint within the epiphysis in a trajectory. It avoids the femoral physis.

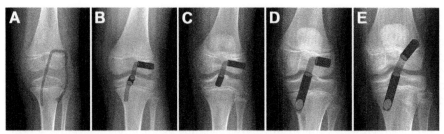

Fig. 4. Radiographs revealing representative images of patients with bone ages of 6 to 14. (*A*) Bone age of 6: Micheli–Kocher intra-articular extra-articular procedure. (*B*) Bone age of 8: Anderson all-epiphyseal procedure, which has been modified. (*C*) Bone age of 10: Ganley–Lawrence all-epiphyseal docking procedure. (*D*) Bone age of 12: Hybrid all-epiphyseal femoral transphyseal tibial procedure. (*E*) Bone age of 14: Transphyseal femoral and tibial reconstruction with soft tissue only at the level of the physis.

portal drilling, outside-in drilling ("2-incision" technique) or an outside-in technique using a retrograde drilling apparatus.[47] The disadvantage of drilling using these methods at more oblique angles, however, is that they can leave the tunnel directed eccentrically through a larger portion of the distal femoral physis and through the perichondral ring (see **Fig. 3**B).[48] With proper intraoperative guidance however, the outside-in techniques can be used to place the femoral tunnel in the anatomic center of the ACL footprint while staying completely within the epiphysis (see **Fig. 3**C).[39,40]

In light of the increased potential risk of growth arrest with standard independent drilling techniques, an all-epiphyseal femoral tunnel may be combined with a traditional transphyseal tibial tunnel. This "hybrid" technique may be appropriately used in older adolescents with a significant amount of growth remaining for surgeons using independent femoral tunnel drilling and has been used by Ganley (**Fig. 4**D).

TREATMENT ALGORITHM BASED ON SKELETAL MATURITY

Based on the rationale presented, the authors offer the following treatment algorithm for selecting a surgical technique in the reconstruction of the ACL in the skeletally immature. The decision for surgery is based on clinical instability, related intra-articular meniscus and cartilage damage, and the patient's activity level and goals to engage in various forms of exercise, as well as the desire to reduce the risk of subsequent meniscal or cartilage damage. After a trial of activity modification, bracing, and rehabilitation, symptomatic patients are candidates for surgical ACL reconstruction (**Fig. 5**). All patients who choose to delay surgical stabilization must understand the risk for ongoing intra-articular damage. Similarly, all patients who choose to proceed with surgical reconstruction must understand the surgical risks and implications, including growth disturbance. Those considering operative treatment must also be mentally and physically prepared to adhere to early and late postoperative protocols that monitor motion, strength, and proprioceptive training.

Using bone age determined by hand radiographs, we stratify our treatment algorithm beginning with prepubescent adolescents ages 3 to 6. We typically use the physeal-sparing combined intra-articular and extra-articular reconstruction technique with autogenous iliotibial band. We also use this technique for slightly older children with less distal femoral epiphyseal bone stock (see **Fig. 4**A). For children ages 7 to 12, we typically use the all-epiphyseal reconstruction technique as described by the authors of this manuscript (see **Fig. 4**C).[40] For smaller patients in this age group,

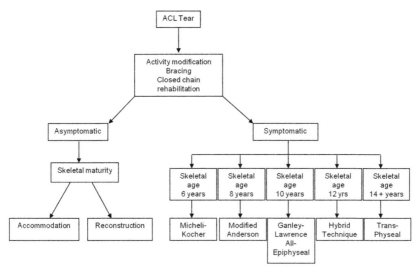

Fig. 5. Treatment algorithm for patients with a ruptured ACL. After a trial of activity modification, bracing, and closed-chain rehabilitation, symptomatic patients are candidates for surgical reconstruction. Prepubescent patients are at greatest risk for growth disturbances, and physeal-sparing techniques such as an all-epiphyseal or combined intra-articular and extra-articular reconstruction are employed. Soft tissue transphyseal reconstruction is performed on older/postpubescent patients.

Ganley uses a modified version of the all-epiphyseal technique (see **Fig. 4**B) if 20 mm of sufficient epiphyseal length is not present to accommodate an epiphyseal retroscrew for tibial fixation. Ganley's modification of the Anderson technique is to perform an all-inside, all epiphyseal procedure using a quadrupled semitendinosis tendon with cortical button fixation at the femur and tibia. For females age 13 and males age 13 to 14, we recommend transphyseal reconstruction using soft tissue graft, usually quadrupled hamstring autograft (see **Fig. 4**E). An alternative reconstruction technique for patients in this age group who still seem to have a significant amount of growth remaining is an all-epiphyseal femoral tunnel centered in the ACL footprint drilled independently either through an all-inside or outside-in technique combined with a transphyseal tibial tunnel using a soft tissue graft (see **Fig. 4**D).

SUMMARY

An increase in the incidence of ACL injuries in skeletally immature athletes has lead to increase in the number of reconstructions performed in this population. Special attention needs to be paid to the needs and concerns of the individual patients and their families. A proper understanding of the physeal anatomy of the distal femur and proximal tibia regarding potential complications from different reconstruction techniques is also required. As techniques evolve, consideration should be given to how these surgeries adhere to established principles related to ACL reconstruction in patients with growth remaining, and how the evolving principles of ACL reconstruction in adults apply to these young patients. We present a treatment algorithm for choosing surgical techniques for ACL reconstruction in the skeletally immature athlete. Ongoing investigation is needed to continue to monitor the intermediate and long-term outcomes of the patients treated with the techniques described. Physicians, patients, and families must share in the decision making regarding the decision for surgery. They must also understand the importance of adhering to rehabilitation and neuromuscular training to promote a safe and timely return to activities and to promote injury prevention.

REFERENCES

1. Clanton TO, DeLee JC, Sanders B, et al. Knee ligament injuries in children. J Bone Joint Surg Am 1979;61:1195–201.
2. DeLee JC, Curtis R. Anterior cruciate ligament insufficiency in children. Clin Orthop Relat Res 1983;172:112–8.
3. Lipscomb AB, Anderson AF. Tears of the anterior cruciate ligament in adolescents. J Bone Joint Surg Am 1986;68:19–28.
4. McCarroll JR, Rettig AC, Shelbourne KD. Anterior cruciate ligament injuries in the young athlete with open physes. Am J Sports Med 1988;16:44–7.
5. Eiskjaer S, Larsen ST, Schmidt MB. The significance of hemarthrosis of the knee in children. Arch Orthop Trauma Surg 1988;107:96–8.
6. Kloeppel-Wirth S, Koltai JL, Dittmer H. Significance of arthroscopy in children with knee joint injuries. Eur J Pediatr Surg 1992;2:169–72.
7. Stanitski CL, Harvell JC, Fu F. Observations on acute knee hemarthrosis in children and adolescents. J Pediatr Orthop 1993;13:506–10.
8. Vahasarja V, Kinnuen P, Serlo W. Arthroscopy of the acute traumatic knee in children. Prospective study of 138 cases. Acta Orthop Scand 1993;64:580–2.
9. Luhmann SJ. Acute traumatic knee effusions in children and adolescents. J Pediatr Orthop 2003;23:199–202.
10. Hennrikus WL. Incidence of tibial spine fractures relative to ACL disruption in the skeletally immature. AAP Annual Meeting 2002.
11. Schaefer RA, Eilert RE, Gillogly SD. Disruption of the anterior cruciate ligament in a 4-year-old child. Orthop Rev 1993;22:725–7.
12. Buckley SL, Barrack RL, Alexander AH. The natural history of conservatively treated partial anterior cruciate ligament tears. Am J Sports Med 1989;17:221–5.
13. Graf BK, Lange RH, Fujisaki CK, et al. Anterior cruciate ligament tears in skeletally immature patients: meniscal pathology at presentation and after attempted conservative treatment. Arthroscopy 1992;8:229–33.
14. Mizuta H, Kubota K, Shiraishi M, et al. The conservative treatment of complete tears of the anterior cruciate ligament in skeletally immature patients. J Bone Joint Surg Br 1995;77:890–4.
15. Janarv PM, Nystrom A, Werner S, et al. Anterior cruciate ligament injuries in skeletally immature patients. J Pediatr Orthop 1996;16:673–7.
16. Pressman AE, Letts RM, Jarvis JG. Anterior cruciate ligament tears in children: an analysis of operative versus nonoperative treatment. J Pediatr Orthop 1997;17:505–11.
17. Kocher MS, Micheli LJ, Zurakowski D, et al. Partial tears of the anterior cruciate ligament in children and adolescents. Am J Sports Med 2002;30:697–703.
18. Aichroth PM, Patel DV, Zorrilla P. The natural history and treatment of rupture of the anterior cruciate ligament in children and adolescents. A prospective review. J Bone Joint Surg Br 2002;84:38–41.
19. Millett PJ, Willis AA, Warren RF. Associated injuries in pediatric and adolescent anterior cruciate ligament tears: does a delay in treatment increase the risk of meniscal tear? Arthroscopy 2002;18:955–9.

20. Arbes S, Resinger C, Vecsei V, et al. The functional outcome of total tears of the anterior cruciate ligament (ACL) in the skeletally immature patient. Int Orthop 2007; 31:471–5.
21. Engebretsen L, Benum P, Sundalsvoll S. Primary suture of the anterior cruciate ligament. A 6-year follow-up of 74 cases. Acta Orthop Scand 1989;60:561–4.
22. Engebretsen L, Svenningsen S, Benum P. Poor results of anterior cruciate ligament repair in adolescence. Acta Orthop Scand 1988;59:684–6.
23. Angel KR, Hall DJ. Anterior cruciate ligament injury in children and adolescents. Arthroscopy 1989;5:197–200.
24. Aronowitz ER, Ganley TJ, Goode JR, et al. Anterior cruciate ligament reconstruction in adolescents with open physes. Am J Sports Med 2000;28:168–75.
25. Lawrence JT, Ganley TJ. Degeneration of the knee joint in skeletally immature patients with an anterior cruciate ligament tear: is there harm in delaying treatment? Paper presented at AOSSM Annual Meeting, Keystone (CO); July 9, 2009.
26. Bhat S, Kanj, W, Lawrence JT, et al. Stochastic decision and cost simulation of early vs. delayed reconstruction of pediatric ACL rupture. Paper presented at AAOS Annual Meeting; San Diego; February 7–11, 2011.
27. Larsen MW, Garrett WE Jr, Delee JC, et al. Surgical management of anterior cruciate ligament injuries in patients with open physes. J Am Acad Orthop Surg 2006;14:736–44.
28. Guzzanti V, Falciglia F, Gigante A, et al. The effect of intra-articular ACL reconstruction on the growth plates of rabbits. J Bone Joint Surg Br 1994;76(6):960–3.
29. Stadelmaier DM, Arnoczky SP, Dodds J, et al. The effect of drilling and soft tissue grafting across open growth plates. A histologic study. Am J Sports Med 1995;23: 431–5.
30. Houle JB, Letts M, Yang J. Effects of a tensioned tendon graft in a bone tunnel across the rabbit physis. Clin Orthop Relat Res 2001;391:275–81.
31. Kocher MS, Saxon HS, Hovis WD, et al. Management and complications of anterior cruciate ligament injuries in skeletally immature patients: survey of the Herodicus Society and The ACL Study Group. J Pediatr Orthop 2002;22:452–7.
32. Koman JD, Sanders JO. Valgus deformity after reconstruction of the anterior cruciate ligament in a skeletally immature patient. A case report. J Bone Joint Surg Am 1999;81:711–5.
33. Frosch KH, Stengel D, Brodhun T, et al. Outcomes and risks of operative treatment of rupture of the anterior cruciate ligament in children and adolescents. Arthroscopy 2010;26:1539–50.
34. Tanner JM, Whitehouse RH. Clinical longitudinal standards for height, weight, height velocity, weight velocity, and stages of puberty. Arch Dis Child 1976;51:170–9.
35. Gruelich WW, Pyle SI. Radiographic atlas of skeletal development of the hand and wrist. 2nd edition. Stanford (CA): Stanford University Press; 1959.
36. Brief LP. Anterior cruciate ligament reconstruction without drill holes. Arthroscopy 1991;7:350–7.
37. Parker AW, Drez D Jr, Cooper JL. Anterior cruciate ligament injuries in patients with open physes. Am J Sports Med 1994;22:44–7.
38. Guzzanti V, Falciglia F, Stanitski CL. Physeal-sparing intraarticular anterior cruciate ligament reconstruction in preadolescents. Am J Sports Med 2003;31:949–53.
39. Anderson AF. Transepiphyseal replacement of the anterior cruciate ligament in skeletally immature patients. A preliminary report. J Bone Joint Surg Am 2003;85A: 1255–63.

40. Lawrence JT, Bowers AL, Belding J, et al. All-epiphyseal anterior cruciate ligament reconstruction in skeletally immature patients. Clin Orthop Relat Res 2010;468: 1971–7.

41. Kocher MS, Garg S, Micheli LJ. Physeal sparing reconstruction of the anterior cruciate ligament in skeletally immature prepubescent children and adolescents. J Bone Joint Surg Am 2005;87:2371–9.

42. Losee RE, Johnson TR, Southwick WO. Anterior subluxation of the lateral tibial plateau. A diagnostic test and operative repair. J Bone Joint Surg Am 1978;60:1015–30.

43. Sankar WN, Carrigan RB, Gregg JR, et al. Anterior cruciate ligament reconstruction in adolescents: a survivorship analysis. Am J Orthop (Belle Mead NJ) 2008;37:47–9.

44. Sankar WN, Wells L, Sennett BJ, et al. Combined anterior cruciate ligament and medial collateral ligament injuries in adolescents. J Pediatr Orthop 2006;26:733–6.

45. Kocher MS, Smith JT, Zoric BJ, et al. Transphyseal anterior cruciate ligament reconstruction in skeletally immature pubescent adolescents. Bone Joint Surg Am 2007;89:2632–9.

46. Abebe ES, Utturkar GM, Taylor DC, et al. The effects of femoral graft placement on in vivo knee kinematics after anterior cruciate ligament reconstruction. J Biomech 2011;44(5):924–9.

47. Abebe ES, Moorman CT 3rd, Dziedzic TS, et al. Femoral tunnel placement during anterior cruciate ligament reconstruction: an in vivo imaging analysis comparing transtibial and 2-incision tibial tunnel-independent techniques. Am J Sports Med 2009;37(10):1904–11.

48. Nelson J, Miller M. Distal femoral physeal implications of an anatomic ACL reconstruction in a skeletally immature soccer player: a case report. J Bone Joint Surg Am 2011;93:e53.

Functional Bracing and Return to Play After Anterior Cruciate Ligament Reconstruction in the Pediatric and Adolescent Patient

Jay C. Albright, MD*, Allison Elizabeth Crepeau, MD

KEYWORDS
- Anterior cruciate ligament reconstruction • Pediatric
- Adolescent • Return to play

Anterior cruciate ligament (ACL) injuries in the pediatric and adolescent population are no longer the rare injury that they once were. Anterior cruciate ligament reconstruction (ACL-R) has become increasing more common in skeletally immature patients because of increased rates of participation in organized sports as well as increased ability to diagnose these injuries. Although younger patients may pursue surgery with the short-term goal of returning to sports quickly, physicians and parents primarily wish to help them stay active, healthy, and safe in terms of minimizing or the risk of further injury. In this article, we will discuss the return-to-play criteria and the use of functional bracing after ACL-R in the pediatric and adolescent population.

RETURN-TO-PLAY CRITERIA

Return to play is not determined by any one criterion. The most common criteria used are: knee (and graft) stability/healing, return of full range of motion, proprioception, strength, and functional strength training that is similar to the unaffected leg.[1]

BIOLOGY OF HEALING

There are multiple graft options available, including autologous bone-patellar tendon-bone, hamstring, and quadriceps tendon, as well as a variety of allograft choices.

No funding sources were used in the preparation of this manuscript.
The corresponding author is a Consultant for Biomet Inc with royalties.
Arnold Palmer Hospital for Children, 83 West Columbia Street, Orlando, FL 32806, USA
* Corresponding author.
E-mail address: Jay.Albright@orlandohealth.com

Clin Sports Med 30 (2011) 811–815
doi:10.1016/j.csm.2011.06.001
0278-5919/11/$ – see front matter © 2011 Elsevier Inc. All rights reserved.

Regardless of graft choice, return to play is limited by the process of graft incorporation and healing.

For the first 4 to 6 weeks, graft stability is solely dependent on initial fixation. Fixation methods have improved dramatically in recent years and now allow for more accelerated rehabilitation protocols. Then, depending on the graft type, bone-to-bone healing or soft tissue–bone incorporation will occur at varying rates. The graft itself will be the weakest part of the construct. Controlled loading and weight bearing are beneficial to graft healing and fiber reorganization. Biologically, grafts are at their weakest point around 4 to 12 weeks postoperatively. This point cannot be emphasized enough, particularly to the young athlete who is usually starting to be pain free and is getting anxious to return to activities. The ACL graft continues to mature for up to a year. However, many studies show that return to play can begin at around 6 months from a graft stability standpoint.[1] The decision is then based on the remaining return-to-play criteria.

RANGE OF MOTION

One of the most common complications of ACL-R is loss of motion; both flexion and extension deficits can occur. Unless a patient has a large bucket-handle meniscus tear or any other type of time-sensitive, motion-limiting injury, surgery should be delayed to allow for resolution of acute inflammation and return of good range of motion. Significantly decreased preoperative range of motion is a risk factor for postoperative loss of motion. Use of a rehabilitation protocol with clearly defined goals and timeframes can be extremely helpful.

Obtaining full extension is one of the primary goals in the early postoperative rehabilitation process. Extension bracing, cryotherapy, and physical therapy can help to decrease the swelling and effusion after surgery and aid in gaining extension. Patella mobilization is also important through the first 8 weeks to achieve flexion goals. Although no one specific protocol has been proven superior, full extension in the first 1 to 2 weeks is a reasonable expectation. We generally recommend aiming for 0 to 90 degrees by 2 to 4 weeks, 0 to 120 degrees by 6 weeks, and 0 to 135 degrees by 8 weeks. We treat motion deficits that persist in this timeframe aggressively. In order avoid iatrogenic fractures or surgical lysis of adhesions we treat persistent motion deficits aggressively. If the patient is unable to obtain 90 degrees of flexion prior to 6 weeks out or 120 degrees 10 weeks out, we perform a manipulation under anesthesia. To avoid iatrogenic fracture or surgical adhesiolysis by performing a manipulation with the patient under anesthesia at around 6 weeks if the patient cannot reach 90 degrees by 10 weeks if the 120-degree goal is not met. Full range of motion is an important criterion, which must be met to proceed with more advanced strength and functional training in the late postoperative rehabilitation process.

STRENGTH

Aside from range of motion, the most important rehabilitative goal for timely return to play is strength. Quadriceps strength is emphasized first because it is necessary for normal gait. One argument for immediate postoperative bracing is to allow early weight bearing while protecting the knee from buckling because of severe quadriceps weakness and inhibition. Postoperative bracing, either with a knee immobilizer or a hinged brace locked in extension, has been shown to have some benefits including decreased swelling, hemarthrosis, and decreased pain. Bracing has not, however, been shown to have any difference in outcomes long term. Once adequate quadriceps strength for ambulation has returned, continued postoperative bracing is unnecessary.

Quad strengthening ideally starts preoperatively and continues throughout the rehabilitation process. Generally we start with isometric quadriceps activation, straight leg raises, and active knee extension. Hamstrings are the ACL agonist, and therefore strengthening of this muscle group is also extremely important. By weeks 5 to 6, the patient may progress to closed chain exercises and then begin to incorporate open chain under the supervision of a physical therapist. Closed chain exercises are generally regarded as safer in the early postoperative period because they minimize shear forces across the knee and simulate more normal proprioceptive stimuli. Quadriceps strength that is at least 85% of the contralateral leg is generally regarded as acceptable for return to play. Looking at the adolescent patient population specifically, Wells et al showed that in the under 20 years of age population, 59% of patients were able to regain greater than 85% quadriceps strength within 6 months.[2] Hamstring strength of 70% to 75% and a hamstring to quadriceps strength ratio that is the same in the uninjured are also commonly used criteria.

PROPRIOCEPTION

Proprioceptive training is another important aspect of postoperative rehabilitation after ACL-R and a necessary consideration for determining return to play. There have been several studies examining the utility of perturbation and neuromuscular training in both ACL-deficient and ACL-R knees. Perturbation training involves forces directed at the affected extremity while standing on an unstable surface, such as a roller board or a wobble board. This type of activity trains the compensatory muscles to act as joint stabilizers.[3] Fitzgerald et al have studied the utility of this type of training in ACL-deficient knees and have shown that incorporation of perturbation training can allow select patients to return to a pre-injury level of activity with absence of giving way episodes.[4,5] Logically then, this type of training can then be applied to both the preoperative and postoperative rehabilitation process of patients undergoing ACL-R. In the preoperative setting, Chmielewski et al showed that 10 perturbation training sessions in patients with acute ACL rupture resulted in knee kinematics that more closely resembled normal knees.[6] The addition of neuromuscular training to a standard strength training–based postoperative rehabilitation protocol did not show any difference in objective strength or functional testing, but did show a significant improvement in subjective knee scores.[7] Although these types of studies have not been applied specifically to the pediatric and adolescent population, they likely would have a similar effect and therefore modifying postoperative rehabilitation to include balance, perturbation, and other proprioceptive training should be considered.

FUNCTIONAL TESTING

Functional testing is often used as an objective measuring tool during rehabilitation after ACL-R. Functional testing can be helpful not only in determining readiness to return to play, but also in determining readiness to progress through a rehabilitation protocol. An alarming number of therapists will judge advancement on a chronologic basis, rather than assessing the progress an individual has made. Using a protocol that incorporates specific objective testing goals can assure the therapist that it is reasonable to delay advancement based on the individual. It must be clear, however, that even if a patient is doing extremely well, it is not advisable to advance patients ahead of schedule in the first 3 months secondary to the basic science of graft healing.

There are many different examples of functional testing, and several of them can be tailored to sport-specific training. Single-leg hop for distance and for vertical height is used to measure power. Single-leg triple hop and other hopping combinations can be used to test both power and endurance. Isokinetic testing is commonly used to measure strength parameters. These guidelines were previously discussed in the section about strength training. Arthrometric data are not commonly used anymore. All of the functional testing data are compared with the uninjured leg, and again, as a general rule, the requirement for return to play should be on the order of 80% to 85%.[1,3,8]

FUNCTIONAL BRACING

Outcomes studies for the use of functional bracing after ACL-R have not been performed strictly for the pediatric and adolescent age group. In fact, until recently, there was no functional brace designed for the pediatric patient available, only adult braces that were modified to fit the smaller and less muscular skeleton. That being said, functional bracing after ALC-R remains controversial. Although often underpowered, numerous studies, including randomized controlled trials, have consistently failed to show any difference in long-term outcomes in range of motion, functional testing, strength, and knee scores.[9,10] The limitation of most of the functional bracing studies is a lack of power. Given that the re-injury rate after ACL-R is very low, the number of patients needed to power the study is exceedingly large, and only one study has been able to show a statistically significant difference in re-injury rates amongst braced versus unbraced skiers.[11] Despite the lack of evidence, many orthopaedic surgeons continue to functionally brace ALC-R knees, particularly during the return-to-play period. A study looking at brace prescription patterns published in 2003 found that 87% of orthopaedic surgeons prescribed functional braces for ACL-R patients.

Benefits of functional bracing may include improved proprioception and increased confidence in the knee during the return-to-play period. We feel that this sense of security, while difficult to quantify scientifically, is of particular benefit to the adolescent population. Additionally, the presence of a functional brace during return to play also serves as a reminder for the patient and players around them that the knee is not normal.

SUMMARY

In conclusion, return-to-play criteria after ACL-R in the pediatric and adolescent population have not been studied extensively, though using the guidelines for adults has proven beneficial. These younger athletes are often extremely anxious to return to their activities, and therefore good communication with the patient, family, and therapist is necessary for a safe and timely rehabilitation program. In general, return to sports should take place at a minimum of 6 months after surgery, though we encourage an objective-based protocol, which should be tailored to each patient depending on the measurable progress. A sense of "readiness" by the patient is not an appropriate indication. Although the assessment of the utility of functional bracing in this population remains scarce and somewhat controversial, it likely still has benefit in this patient population.

REFERENCES

1. Honkamp NJ, Shen W, Okeke N, et al. Rehabilitation considerations in anterior cruciate ligament injuries in the adult. In: DeLee JC, Drez D Jr, Miller MD, editors. DeLee and Drez's orthopaedic sports medicine. 3rd edition. Philadelphia: Saunders; 2009. p. 1670–6.

2. Wells L, Dyke JA, Albaugh J, et al. Adolescent anterior cruciate ligament reconstruction: a retrospective analysis of quadriceps strength recovery and return to full activity after surgery. J Pediatr Orthop 2009;29:486–9.

3. Pezzullo DJ, Fadale P. Current controversies in rehabilitation after anterior cruciate ligament reconstruction. Sports Med Arthrosc Rev 2010;18(1):43–7.

4. Fitzgerald GK, Axe M, Snyder-Mackler L. Proposed practice guidelines for nonoperative ACL rehabilitation of physically active individuals. J Orthop Sports Phys Ther 2000;30:194–203.

5. Fitzgerald GK, Axe M, Snyder-Mackler L. The efficacy of perturbation training in nonoperative anterior cruciate ligament rehabilitation programs for physically active individuals. Phys Ther 2000;80(2):128–40.

6. Chmielewski T, Hurd W, Rudolph K, et al. Perturbation training improves knee kinematics and reduces muscle co-contraction after complete unilateral ligament rupture. Phys Ther 2005;85(8):740–54.

7. Risberg A, Holm I, Myklebust G, et al. Neuromuscular training versus strength training during first 6 months after anterior ligament reconstruction: a randomized clinical trial. Phys Ther 2007;87:737–50.

8. Cascio BM, Culp L, Cosgarea AJ. Return to play after anterior cruciate ligament reconstruction. Clin Sports Med 2004;23:395–408.

9. Wright RW, Fetzer GB. Bracing after ACL reconstruction: a systematic review. Clin Orthop Relat Res 2007;455:162–8.

10. McDevitt ER, Taylor DC, Miller MD, et al. Functional bracing after anterior cruciate ligament reconstruction: a prospective, randomized, multicenter study. Am J Sports Med 2004;32(8):1887–92.

11. Sterett W, Briggs K, Farley T, et al. Effect of functional bracing on knee injury in skiers with anterior cruciate ligament reconstruction: a prospective cohort study. Am J Sports Med 2006;34:1581–5.

Anterior Cruciate Ligament Reconstruction Rehabilitation in the Pediatric Population

Lisa M. Kruse, MD, Benjamin L. Gray, MD, Rick W. Wright, MD*

KEYWORDS
- Anterior cruciate ligament • Rehabilitation • Pediatric
- Reconstruction

Anterior cruciate ligament (ACL) reconstruction rehabilitation in the pediatric population offers some similarities and a few differences compared with adult ACL reconstruction rehabilitation. Many of the fundamental principles remain applicable to the pediatric population. The challenge for the orthopedic surgeon performing ACL reconstruction in this population is the knowledge that of all of the patients that they interface with this group has the highest likelihood to return to a high level of activity. Thus, their expectations are to have an outstanding outcome after this procedure. An understanding of this can help the physician to challenge the patient to assist in obtaining these results by actively participating in their rehabilitation.

SURGICAL FACTORS

Surgical factors at the time of reconstruction can impact the patient's ability to appropriately rehabilitate their ACL reconstructed knee. These include surgical timing, graft material, graft position, graft tension, and graft fixation. Surgical timing refers to allowing the knee to calm down and regain full extension and flexion before reconstruction. Graft material implies that a graft of appropriate strength is utilized that will not deform during the forces seen while rehabilitating the knee. If a graft is malpositioned, excessive force to regain motion may stretch the graft. The ACL graft must be appropriately tensioned and not excessively loose to restore appropriate kinematics and allow appropriate motion to be regained. The fixation for the graft must be sufficiently strong to allow early motion without risk of loss of fixation of the graft. Graft and surgical technique choice are impacted by patients with open physes. This may also have an impact on rehabilitation but no research is published in this area.

Department of Orthopaedic Surgery, Washington University School of Medicine, #1 Barnes Hospital Plaza, Suite 11300 West Pavilion, St Louis, MO 63110, USA
* Corresponding author.
E-mail address: wright@wudosis.wustl.edu

Clin Sports Med 30 (2011) 817–824
doi:10.1016/j.csm.2011.06.005
0278-5919/11/$ – see front matter © 2011 Elsevier Inc. All rights reserved.
sportsmed.theclinics.com

REHABILITATION FUNDAMENTALS

Many of the aspects of ACL reconstruction rehabilitation have been studied in a research setting. Some aspects are intuitive and have become fundamentals without true scientific evidence. In the modern era of ACL rehabilitation, early motion has become a guiding principle. Although this has not been necessarily studied by a randomized trial, surgeons noted improved results when they stopped cast immobilization and started early range of motion work. Based on this, patients should begin range of motion work within the first week after their ACL reconstruction.

Wright and colleagues[1,2] in 2008 published 2 systematic reviews of the level 1 and 2 clinical trials that assessed aspects of ACL reconstruction rehabilitation. A total of 54 studies were included in these reviews. This formed the basis for development of the Multi-Center Orthopedic Outcome Network ACL rehabilitation protocol. We review the findings from these systematic reviews and then present new data that has arisen since these reviews were performed in 2005.

Continuous Passive Motion

Continuous passive motion (CPM) was evaluated by 4 studies in systematic review before 2005 and found to provide no improved range of motion or outcome and thus was felt not to be indicated based on lack of scientific evidence indicating its use and lack of potential insurance approval and cost to the patient. Since the systematic review, an additional study investigated the use of CPM and its effects on proprioception; no clinically significant difference was found.[3] This agrees with prior studies in that it does not support the use of CPM.

Weight Bearing

Immediate weight bearing after ACL reconstruction has been evaluated in 1 trial.[4] This study demonstrated a decrease of patellofemoral pain after reconstruction from 35% to 8% with early full weight bearing. Thus, it is appropriate for patients to progress to full weight bearing as quickly as possible after routine ACL reconstruction.

Bracing

In the prior systematic review, 11 studies evaluated a variety of postoperative bracing parameters.[5] No study demonstrated improved range of motion, increased ease of obtaining extension, increased safety, or decreased complications with bracing. The control groups in no study demonstrated a worse outcome with regard to any rehabilitation parameter. After the systematic review, a 5-year follow-up of braced versus non-braced patients continued to show no difference in outcomes.[6] Two additional studies compared different types of bracing to functional knee braces. Use of a neoprene sleeve did not alter outcomes, although patients reported a subjective higher confidence level in the brace.[7] A knee immobilizer used immediately postoperatively did not affect pain scores or use of analgesic during the first 2 weeks after surgery.[8] A soft, fluid-filled brace decreased effusion, swelling, extensor mechanism deficit (by approximately 1°) and patient-measured outcomes compared with the hard brace.[9] Based on this, we cannot recommend postoperative bracing as necessary after ACL reconstruction.

Home-Based Rehabilitation

Four studies included in prior systematic reviews evaluated home-based rehabilitation and found that, in the motivated patient, appropriate rehabilitation milestones can be met and completed with decreased outpatient-based physical therapy intervention. A caveat exists in the pediatric population, where the physician should closely monitor the patient to make sure that they are appropriately motivated and achieving their rehabilitation goals if not under the auspices of a physical therapist. Additional 2- to 4-year follow-up of 1 study included in the previous systematic review found similar outcomes between home-based and therapist-assisted rehabilitation.[10] An additional study comparing hospital-based therapy with guided home-based therapy found improved knee scores at 6 months in the hospital-based therapy group, but the trend reversed and the home-based rehabilitation group had a greater improvement in knee scores at 12 months.[11] We recommend that rehabilitation in pediatric patients continue to be closely monitored by a physician if they are not participating in formal outpatient physical therapy.

Hamstring and Quadriceps Strengthening and Motion

The original systematic review found that straight leg raises for quadriceps strengthening is safe and can be started immediately postoperatively without increased risk of graft laxity or stretching. Since the systematic review was performed, a number of studies have evaluated the timing of rehabilitation. One compared 3 days with 2 weeks of immobilization after ACL reconstruction with multistrand hamstring graft, and found no difference between the groups with regard to laxity, joint position sense, or quadriceps strength.[12] Shaw and co-workers[13] found that straight leg raises and isometric quadriceps contraction in first 2 postoperative weeks had higher initial pain scores, fewer problems with sports, and no increase in average knee laxity.[13] Full active and passive extension training immediately postoperatively (compared with 4 weeks postoperatively) does not result in increased knee laxity.[14] Isokinetic hamstring strengthening exercises can be started at postoperative week 3 with no negative impact on knee function.[15] One study compared tibial and femoral tunnel size on computed tomography in patients who received either immediate brace-free rehabilitation or 2 weeks of immobilization and no strengthening until 6 weeks; there was significantly increased size of both femoral and tibial tunnels with immediate rehabilitation, although this difference was not clinically significant.[16] Gerber and associates[17] compared 12 weeks of eccentric strengthening with concentric strengthening starting 3 weeks postoperatively in 2 studies. No differences were noted between groups with regard to stability at 26 weeks, but patients in eccentric strengthening group demonstrated greater quadriceps strength and hopping distance.[17] Magnetic resonance imaging at both 3 weeks and 1 year showed increased volume and cross-sectional area of gluteal and quadriceps muscles and continued increase in strength and hopping distance in eccentric strengthening group.[18] We recommend the inclusion of eccentric exercises as part of the rehabilitation program after ACL reconstruction; studies have shown that these exercises can safely be started at 3 weeks postoperatively.

Accelerated Rehabilitation

A study by Beynnon and colleagues[19] found no difference in knee laxity, clinical satisfaction, or activity in accelerated versus non-accelerated rehabilitation after 1 year.[19] A few studies have tried to evaluate accelerated rehabilitation, but accelerated has typically meant 6 months versus a truly accelerated return of the athletes to play at 3 to 4 months. It seems that a 6-month–based rehabilitation protocol remains safe and effective and continues to be the norm.

Open- Versus Closed-Chain Kinetic Rehabilitation

Despite its perceived importance for ACL rehabilitation, only 5 randomized trials comparing open- with closed-chain kinetic rehabilitation methods were found in the prior systematic review. Three of these trials involve the same patient population studied at 6 weeks postoperatively and thus conclusions from these 3 studies may not be appropriately applied to a 6-month outcome. After the systematic review, an additional randomized, controlled trial assessed open- and closed-chain kinetic exercises starting 8 weeks after surgery, and found no differences in knee laxity or leg function.[20] Based on the studies that have been performed, it seems safe to add open-chain kinetic strengthening 6 weeks postoperatively. It may be safe earlier, but there is not strong evidence to support this. Thus, closed-kinetic chain rehabilitation exercises are recommended until 6 weeks have passed.

Proprioception and Vibration Training

A randomized, controlled trial by Cooper and colleagues[21] compared proprioceptive and balance training with traditional strengthening after ACL reconstruction. The outcomes were similar, except that the strengthening group had higher scores on Cincinnati knee rating and patient specific functional scale. Vibratory stimulation was found to improve postural stability and peak torques,[22] as well as in proprioception and balance in athletes using a biodex stability system.[23] (There is no evidence that proprioception or vibration training causes harm after ACL reconstruction, and it is likely a beneficial supplement to traditional rehabilitation.

Neuromuscular training (balance exercises, dynamic joint stability exercises, agility drills, plyometric exercises, and sport-specific exercises) was compared with strength training (strengthening of quadriceps, hamstrings, gluteal, and gastrocnemius muscles) in 1 study. It found that the neuromuscular training group had improved knee function and decreased pain during activity, whereas the strength training group had improved hamstring strength.[24] Initially at 6 months, the neuromuscular training group had significantly improved Cincinnati knee and VAS score compared with the strength training group,[25] but at 2 years there were no differences in the Cincinnati knee score.[24] Given these results, both neuromuscular and strength training can be included in rehabilitation after ACL reconstruction.

Neuromuscular Electrical Stimulation

Fourteen studies evaluated neuromuscular electrical stimulation and were included in the original systematic review. These used a variety of devices, parameters, and settings. Conclusions regarding this group are difficult to make; however, some general conclusions can be made. A high-intensity setting must be applied early in the postoperative period and it seems that home-based units do not provide enough power to successfully improve quadriceps strength. A recent systematic review of neuromuscular electrical stimulation on quadriceps strength including 8 studies concluded that it may improve quadriceps strength, but the effect on functional performance and patient-oriented outcomes is inconclusive.[26] Neuromuscular electrical stimulation may help to achieve improved quadriceps strength, but we have not found it to be a requirement or necessary for successful ACL reconstruction rehabilitation. Thus, we have left it up to the discretion of the physical therapist.

Supplements

Two studies evaluated the effects of various supplements on ACL rehabilitation. Huang and colleagues[27] studied the early effects of hyaluronic acid injections after

ACL reconstruction; groups receiving hyaluronic acid injections at 8 or 12 weeks demonstrated improvement in ambulation speed and muscle peak torque.[27] Barker and co-workers[28] studied the effect of vitamin E and C supplementation and found that it did not improve strength. Based on these data, we do not recommend supplementation or injections at this time.

Miscellaneous Studies

A few niche studies evaluated some very discreet aspects of ACL rehabilitation. Water-based therapy may decrease swelling. Slide board exercises may be added in the 6- to 8-week postoperative time frame without risk of injury. Stair climber is as safe as stationary cycling and can be added at the 4- to 6-week time frame. One-legged (unaffected leg) stationary cycling combined with traditional rehabilitation showed decreased cardiac deconditioning in soccer players after 6 weeks.[29] Specific programs aimed at running retraining are well-tolerated, but provide no additional benefit with regard to strength, knee laxity, or Lysholm knee scores.[30] Biophysical stimulation (magnetic field) studied in a 60-patient randomized, controlled trial demonstrated faster recovery (per SF-36) and less limitation in passive range of motion.[31] One underpowered study evaluated the effect of video modeling on self-efficacy during rehabilitation as well as rehabilitation outcomes. They found that patients in the modeling group had lower preoperative expectations of pain, greater self-efficacy at discharge for rehabilitation, and better International Knee Documentation Committee functional outcome scores.[32]

Table 1
Postoperative physical therapy

Phase	Timing	Components
1	Immediately postoperatively	Weight bearing
		Range of motion 0°–90°
		Strengthening with closed chain exercises, straight leg raise, and isometric quadriceps exercises
2	Week 3	Neuromuscular training—balance
		Eccentric quadriceps strengthening
		Isokinetic hamstring strengthening
		Cycling
3	Week 6	Open-chain kinetic exercises
4	Week 9	Increase weight in closed- and open-chain kinetic
		Neuromuscular plyometric exercises, jumping 2 leg to 1 leg
Phase 5	Week 12	Begin jogging
Phase 6	Week 15	Jumping, agility training and sport specific training
Return to sport criteria	6 Months postoperatively	No pain or swelling
		Full range of motion
		Quadriceps strength 85% contralateral side
		Hop test 85% contralateral side
		Tolerating sport specific activities and agility training

SUMMARY

Although we assume fundamentals of rehabilitation after pediatric ACL reconstruction are similar to that for adults, no studies specifically address rehabilitation after ACL reconstruction in the pediatric patient. Pediatric patients are more likely to expect to return to a high activity level after ACL reconstruction, so it is important to monitor their rehabilitation closely. Although additional modalities in rehabilitation after ACL reconstruction require more research, they have not been shown to have a detrimental effect on graft success and may safely be implemented into a rehabilitation protocol.

Based on the studies presented earlier we recommend the following guidelines for rehabilitation of pediatric patient after ACL reconstruction.

- Before surgery preoperative range of motion should be full and knee should be calm.[33]
- Neither CPM or bracing is necessary in adults and this may also be the case for children as well. There are, however, no current strictly pediatric studies available for review.
- Rehabilitation may effectively be done as a home-based program, although pediatric patients may benefit from further supervision.
- Postoperative physical therapy should emphasize quadriceps strengthening, flexion, and return of gait (**Table 1**).

With the increase in pediatric ACL injuries and their expectation to return to high-level activities, specific studies investigating rehabilitation in pediatric populations will be exceedingly valuable in the future.

REFERENCES

1. Wright RW, Preston E, Fleming BC, et al. A systematic review of anterior cruciate ligament reconstruction rehabilitation: part II: open versus closed kinetic chain exercises, neuromuscular electrical stimulation, accelerated rehabilitation, and miscellaneous topics. J Knee Surg 2008;21:225–34.
2. Wright RW, Preston E, Fleming BC, et al. A systematic review of anterior cruciate ligament reconstruction rehabilitation: part I: continuous passive motion, early weight bearing, postoperative bracing, and home-based rehabilitation. J Knee Surg 2008; 21:217–24.
3. Friemert B, Bach C, Schwarz W, et al. Benefits of active motion for joint position sense. Knee Surg Sports Traumatol Arthrosc 2006;14:564–70.
4. Timm KE. The clinical and cost-effectiveness of two different programs for rehabilitation following ACL reconstruction. J Orthop Sports Phys Ther 1997;25:43–8.
5. Wright RW, Fetzer GB. Bracing after ACL reconstruction: a systematic review. Clin Orthop Relat Res 2007;455:162–8.
6. Harilainen A, Sandelin J. Post-operative use of knee brace in bone-tendon-bone patellar tendon anterior cruciate ligament reconstruction: 5-year follow-up results of a randomized prospective study. Scand J Med Sci Sports 2006;16:14–8.
7. Birmingham TB, Bryant DM, Giffin JR, et al. A randomized controlled trial comparing the effectiveness of functional knee brace and neoprene sleeve use after anterior cruciate ligament reconstruction. Am J Sports Med 2008;36:648–55.
8. Hiemstra LA, Heard SM, Sasyniuk TM, et al. Knee immobilization for pain control after a hamstring tendon anterior cruciate ligament reconstruction: a randomized clinical trial. Am J Sports Med 2009;37:56–64.

9. Mayr HO, Hochrein A, Hein W, et al. Rehabilitation results following anterior cruciate ligament reconstruction using a hard brace compared to a fluid-filled soft brace. Knee 2010;17:119–26.

10. Grant JA, Mohtadi NG. Two- to 4-year follow-up to a comparison of home versus physical therapy-supervised rehabilitation programs after anterior cruciate ligament reconstruction. Am J Sports Med 2010;38:1389–94.

11. Revenas A, Johansson A, Leppert J. A randomized study of two physiotherapeutic approaches after knee ligament reconstruction. Adv Physiother 2009;11:30–41.

12. Ito Y, Deie M, Adachi N, et al. A prospective study of 3-day versus 2-week immobilization period after anterior cruciate ligament reconstruction. Knee 2007;14:34–8.

13. Shaw T, Williams MT, Chipchase LS. Do early quadriceps exercises affect the outcome of ACL reconstruction? A randomised controlled trial. Aust J Physiother 2005;51:9–17.

14. Isberg J, Faxen E, Brandsson S, et al. Early active extension after anterior cruciate ligament reconstruction does not result in increased laxity of the knee. Knee Surg Sports Traumatol Arthrosc 2006;14:1108–15.

15. Sekir U, Gur H, Akova B. Early versus late start of isokinetic hamstring-strengthening exercise after anterior cruciate ligament reconstruction with patellar tendon graft. Am J Sports Med 2010;38:492–500.

16. Vadala A, Iorio R, De Carli A, et al. The effect of accelerated, brace free, rehabilitation on bone tunnel enlargement after ACL reconstruction using hamstring tendons: a CT study. Knee Surg Sports Traumatol Arthrosc 2007;15:365–71.

17. Gerber JP, Marcus RL, Dibble LE, et al. Effects of early progressive eccentric exercise on muscle structure after anterior cruciate ligament reconstruction. J Bone Joint Surg Am 2007;89:559–70.

18. Gerber JP, Marcus RL, Dibble LE, et al. Effects of early progressive eccentric exercise on muscle size and function after anterior cruciate ligament reconstruction: a 1-Year follow-up study of a Randomized Clinical Trial. Phys Ther 2009;89:51–9.

19. Beynnon BD, Uh BS, Johnson RJ, et al. Rehabilitation after anterior cruciate ligament reconstruction: a prospective, randomized, double-blind comparison of programs administered over 2 different time intervals. Am J Sports Med 2005;33:347–59.

20. Perry MC, Morrissey MC, King JB, et al. Effects of closed versus open kinetic chain knee extensor resistance training on knee laxity and leg function in patients during the 8- to 14-week post-operative period after anterior cruciate ligament reconstruction. Knee Surg Sports Traumatol Arthrosc 2005;13:357–69.

21. Cooper RL, Taylor NF, Feller JA. A randomised controlled trial of proprioceptive and balance training after surgical reconstruction of the anterior cruciate ligament. Res Sports Med 2005;13:217–30.

22. Brunetti O, Filippi GM, Lorenzini M, et al. Improvement of posture stability by vibratory stimulation following anterior cruciate ligament reconstruction. Knee Surg Sports Traumatol Arthrosc 2006;14:1180–7.

23. Moezy A, Olyaei G, Hadian M, et al. A comparative study of whole body vibration training and conventional training on knee proprioception and postural stability after anterior cruciate ligament reconstruction. Br J Sports Med 2008;42:373–8.

24. Risberg MA, Holm I. The long-term effect of 2 postoperative rehabilitation programs after anterior cruciate ligament reconstruction: a randomized controlled clinical trial with 2 years of follow-up. Am J Sports Med 2009;37:1958–66.

25. Risberg MA, Holm I, Myklebust G, et al. Neuromuscular training versus strength training during first 6 months after anterior cruciate ligament reconstruction: a randomized clinical trial. Phys Ther 2007;87:737–50.

26. Kim KM, Croy T, Hertel J, et al. Effects of neuromuscular electrical stimulation after anterior cruciate ligament reconstruction on quadriceps strength, function, and patient-oriented outcomes: a systematic review. J Orthop Sports Phys Ther 2010;40: 383–91.

27. Huang MH, Yang RC, Chou PH. Preliminary effects of hyaluronic acid on early rehabilitation of patients with isolated anterior cruciate ligament reconstruction. Clin J Sport Med 2007;17:242–50.

28. Barker T, Leonard SW, Hansen J, et al. Vitamin E and C supplementation does not ameliorate muscle dysfunction after anterior cruciate ligament surgery. Free Radic Biol Med 2009;47:1611–8.

29. Olivier N, Weissland T, Legrand R, et al. The effect of a one-leg cycling aerobic training program during the rehabilitation period in soccer players with anterior cruciate ligament reconstruction. Clin J Sport Med 2010;20:28–33.

30. Dauty M, Menu P, Dubois C. Effects of running retraining after knee anterior cruciate ligament reconstruction. Ann Phys Rehabil Med 2010;53:150–61.

31. Benazzo F, Zanon G, Pederzini L, et al. Effects of biophysical stimulation in patients undergoing arthroscopic reconstruction of anterior cruciate ligament: prospective, randomized and double blind study. Knee Surg Sports Traumatol Arthrosc 2008;16: 595–601.

32. Maddison R, Prapavessis H, Clatworthy M. Modeling and rehabilitation following anterior cruciate ligament reconstruction. Ann Behav Med 2006;31:89–98.

33. Halinen J, Lindahl J, Hirvensalo E. Range of motion and quadriceps muscle power after early surgical treatment of acute combined anterior cruciate and grade-III medial collateral ligament injuries. A prospective randomized study. J Bone Joint Surg Am 2009;91:1305–12.

Does an In-Season Only Neuromuscular Training Protocol Reduce Deficits Quantified by the Tuck Jump Assessment?

Madelyn F. Klugman,[a,b] Jensen L. Brent,CSCS,[a]
Gregory D. Myer, PhD, CSCS,[a,c,d,e],* Kevin R. Ford, PhD,[a,c]
Timothy E. Hewett, PhD,[a,c,d]

KEYWORDS
- Anterior cruciate ligament injury • Knee
- Drop vertical jump landing • Young athletes
- Injury Risk Assessment • Neuromuscular training outcomes

Adolescent female soccer players are 4 to 6 times more likely to sustain an anterior cruciate ligament (ACL) injury than are male soccer players.[1,2] This sex disparity may be caused by decreased neuromuscular control during the execution of sports movements, particularly in landing and pivoting movements. This results in lower limb mechanics, which may increase ACL injury risk.[3,4,5] Several injury prevention programs have been developed in order to reduce the risk of ACL as well as other lower extremity injuries.[6-16]

The authors would like to acknowledge funding support from National Institutes of Health (grants R01-AR049735, R01-AR055563, and R01-AR056259).
The Cincinnati Children's Hospital Medical Center and Byram Hill High School Institutional Review Boards approved this study.
[a] Division of Sports Medicine, Cincinnati Children's Hospital Medical Center, 3333 Burnet Avenue, Cincinnati, OH 45229, USA
[b] Byram Hills High School, Armonk, NY 10504, USA
[c] Department of Pediatrics and Orthopaedic Surgery, College of Medicine, University of Cincinnati, Cincinnati, OH 45221, USA
[d] Departments of Physiology and Cell Biology, Orthopaedic Surgery, Family Medicine and Biomedical Engineering, The Ohio State University Sports Health & Performance Institute, The Ohio State University, Columbus, OH 43221, USA
[e] Departments of Athletic Training, Sports Orthopaedics, and Pediatric Science, Rocky Mountain University of Health Professions, Provo, UT 84606, USA
* Corresponding author: Division of Sports Medicine Cincinnati, Children's Hospital Medical Center, 3333 Burnet Avenue, Cininnati, OH 45229.
E-mail address: greg.myer@chmcc.org

Clin Sports Med 30 (2011) 825–840
doi:10.1016/j.csm.2011.07.001
0278-5919/11/$ – see front matter © 2011 Elsevier Inc. All rights reserved.

One major factor differentiating neuromuscular training programs is the varied programming within the yearly calendar. Performing the training in-season or preseason may have varying effects on injury risk throughout the competitive season. If preseason training is omitted, there is potentially a greater injury risk in the early season, while the consequences of not performing in-season training may manifest themselves as the season continues and the potential benefits of the preseason training becomes negligible.

In-season training is characterized by shorter, less intensive training as systemic fatigue can hinder sports performance.[7] The most effective and efficient programs in both types of protocols should include four essential components: balance, biofeedback, strength, and plyometric exercises.[17] In a meta-analysis of ACL injury prevention training studies, Hewett and colleagues concluded that an in-season protocol alone is likely the most cost-effective; however, the decrease in injury risk may not manifest itself until much later in the season due to the reduced intensity of the training.[18] Nevertheless, several studies have tested the influence of in-season training and have had positive results. Gilchrist and colleagues[7] indicated that an on-field warm-up program significantly reduced ACL injury rates, Pollard and coworkers[19] demonstrated that joint kinematics and kinetics were improved after an in-season intervention, and Zebis and colleagues[20] reported increased EMG activity in the medial hamstrings. The authors proposed this increased activity would reduce dynamic knee valgus and the resultant injury risk.[21]

Prospective measures of high dynamic knee valgus (ie, knee abduction moment) during landing predict ACL injury risk in young female athletes.[21] In addition, a large-scale prospective study found that military cadets who sustained ACL injuries demonstrated knee landing mechanics related to these coronal plane knee deficits.[22] Several investigations have demonstrated that female athletes more often exhibit excessive coronal plane load and motion landing mechanics compared to males during landing and pivoting movements.[3–5,23–29] In validation of theses laboratory findings, females often demonstrate knee landing alignments associated with high knee abduction load at the time of injury.[30–32]

The aforementioned studies required the use of expensive, 3-dimensional motion capture equipment to evaluate and predict ACL injury risk by tracking kinetics and kinematics. The cost of using 3-dimensional motion analysis to measure kinetics and kinematics can be in the range of $1000 per athlete per test.[33] These costs easily exceed the budgets of most high school athletic programs. In addition, Myer and coworkers recently demonstrated that laboratory-based injury risk identification techniques can be successfully applied to clinical practice.[33–35] The current study seeks to expand on this concept through the implementation of a field-based evaluation to test the effects of in-season neuromuscular training.[36,37] This study implemented a "clinician-friendly" plyometric assessment that requires substantially less equipment and personnel than 3-dimensional motion analysis. In this assessment, athletes performed consecutive tuck jumps for 10 seconds while the clinician subsequently identifies any of 10 possible deficiencies associated with neuromuscular risk factors shown through motion analysis (eg, "lower extremity valgus at landing").[36,37] Each athlete's baseline performance was then compared to their post-training performances. An athlete who was identified with at least 6 of the 10 risk factors in the tuck jump would theoretically receive high-intensity training options, since neuromuscular interventions best benefit high-risk athletes.[36,37] The purpose of this study was to identify the effects of an in-season warm-up training program on young female

Table 1 Subject demographics			
Group	Mean Age (y)	Mean Height (cm)	Mean Mass (kg)
In-season neuromuscular training (IN) group (n = 15)	14.1 (SD, 0.4)	161.4 (SD, 5.0)	50.4 (SD, 5.7)
Control (CTRL) (n = 34)	14.7 (SD, 1.0)	163.7 (SD, 5.7)	57.0 (SD, 9.2)

soccer players. The hypothesis tested was that the ACL prevention training program included with an in-season soccer program would demonstrate increased improvement in the Tuck Jump Assessment (TJA) scores at postseason follow-up testing relative to standard in-season soccer training.

METHODS
Subjects

Female high school varsity and junior varsity soccer players from two Westchester County, New York, school districts volunteered to participate in the study. The in-season neuromuscular training group (IN) consisted of 15 subjects, and 34 subjects from another high school soccer team formed the control group (CTRL). Subject height, mass, age, and descriptions of previous injuries were recorded for each subject (Table 1). Parents or guardians signed informed consent forms approved by the institutional review board, and assent from the child participants was obtained prior to study participation.

Testing Procedures

Both groups were tested before and after the soccer season. Standard camcorders were mounted on tripods, providing independent sagittal and frontal plane views of the subject. Subjects were shown a video presentation and a live demonstration of correct tuck jump technique. Subjects were then allowed to ask questions and were provided with unlimited practice time. Subjects were instructed to place their feet on markings that were 35 cm apart. Subjects completed consecutive tuck jumps for 10 seconds as described.[36,37]

Videos were imported into iMovie 6.0.3 (Apple, Cupertino, CA, USA), synchronized, and merged into split-screen using a plug-in (SplitScreen & PiP, StupendousSoftware. com) Two raters, blinded to both the training status and training type, subsequently evaluated for the presence of criteria-based biomechanical deficits shown in videos provided in a random order. These criteria have been previously reported as potential underlying contributors to increased risk of knee injury in female athletes (Fig. 1).[36,37] To determine an athlete's preseason and post season score, their individual score was averaged between the 2 raters.

Neuromuscular Intervention

The CTRL group received no intervention and continued their regular in-season routine. This routine was a standard soccer warm-up that included light jogging and static stretching. The IN group received a neuromuscular intervention that was developed using previously published protocols and further adapted for this study (Table 2).[38,39] The protocol implemented with the IN group consisted of an abbreviated protocol of five, two-week progressions of 6 exercises: single-leg anterior

Tuck Jump Assessment	Pre	Mid	Post	Comments
Knee and Thigh Motion				
① Lower extremity valgus at landing	☐	☐	☐	
② Thighs do not reach parallel (peak of jump)	☐	☐	☐	
③ Thighs not equal side-to-side (during flight)	☐	☐	☐	
Foot Position During Landing				
④ Foot placement not shoulder width apart	☐	☐	☐	
⑤ Foot placement not parallel (front to back)	☐	☐	☐	
⑥ Foot contact timing not equal	☐	☐	☐	
7. Excessive landing contact noise	☐	☐	☐	
Plyometric Technique				
8. Pause between jumps	☐	☐	☐	
9. Technique declines prior to 10 seconds	☐	☐	☐	
10. Does not land in same footprint (excessive in-flight motion)	☐	☐	☐	
	Total ____	Total ____	Total ____	

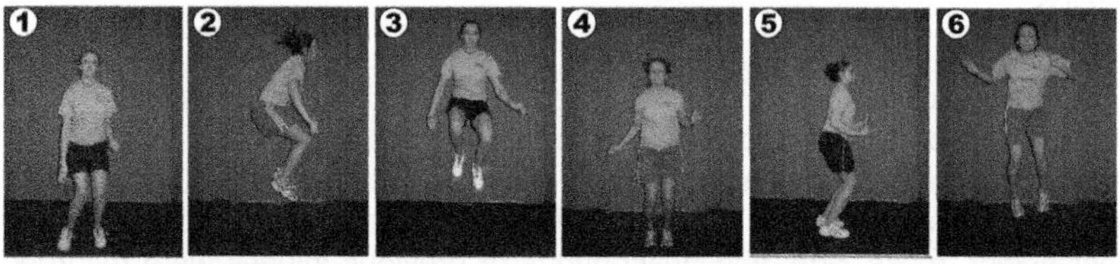

Fig. 1. Tuck Jump Assessment (TJA) tool can be used to score deficits during a jumping and landing sequence movement. To perform the TJA, the athlete is instructed to start in the athletic position with her feet shoulder-width apart (on line marked 35 cm apart). She is instructed to initiate the jump with a slight crouch downward while she extends her arms behind her. She then swings her arms forward as she simultaneously jumps straight up and pulls her knees up as high as possible. At the highest point of the jump, the athlete is instructed to pull her thighs parallel to the ground. When landing, the athlete should immediately begin the next tuck jump. Encourage the athlete to land softly, using a toe to mid-foot rocker landing and land in the same footprint with each jump. The athlete is instructed to perform the tuck jump exercise for 10 seconds and should be instructed to not continue this jump if they demonstrate a sharp decline in technique during the allotted time frame. (*Reproduced from* Myer GD, Ford KR, et al. Tuck jump assessment for reducing anterior cruciate ligament injury risk. Athletic Therapy Today 2008;13(5):39-44; with permission.)

progression, single-leg rotary progression, unanticipated hop-to-stabilization, hop-to-stabilization and reach, tuck jump progression, and hamstring strength progression. Progressions were presented to the coaching staff in the form of a training manual (**Table 1**). The coach was instructed to give continuous verbal feedback to the subjects during and after the intervention and were given the common verbalizations and visualizations “land light as a feather,” “on your toes,” “straight as an arrow,” “shock absorber” and “recoil like a spring” as suggestions.[16,40]

Statistics

A mixed-design (2×2; group $\times$ time) repeated-measures ANOVA was used to test the interaction and main effects of group (neuromuscular intervention versus standard soccer training) and time (preseason/training versus in-season/training) on TJA scores. Statistical analyses were conducted in SPSS (Version 17.0; SPSS, Chicago, IL, USA). Statistical significance was established a priori at $P \leq .05$.

Table 2
In-season training protocol

Exercise Name	Description Phase 1 (Weeks 1-2)	Reps	Sets
1. Single Leg Anterior Progression Step-hold	The athlete takes a quick step forward and continues by balancing in a deep hold position on the leg onto which she stepped.	8	2 (1 per side)
2. Single Leg Rotary Progression Single-leg 90-degree hold	The athlete starts in a semicrouched position on the single limb being trained The jump should focus on attaining maximum height while maintaining good form upon landing. During the flight phase, the athlete should rotate 90 degrees. The landing occurs on the same leg and should be performed with deep knee flexion. The landing should be held for a minimum of 3 seconds to be counted as successful. Coach this jump with care to protect the athlete from injury. Start the athlete with a submaximal effort so she can experience the difficulty of the jump. Continue to increase the intensity of the jump as the athlete improves her ability to stick and hold the final landing. Have the athlete keep her focus away from her feet to help protect too much forward lean.	8	2 (1 per side)
3. Unanticipated Hop to Stabilization	Place 9 cones 18 inches apart. The coach will shout a sequence of 9 numbers from 1 to 9. Athletes can use any type of hop (anterior-posterior, medial-lateral, or a combination) to get to corresponding cones. Allow 5 seconds per hop.	9	3
4. Hop to Stabilization and Reach	From starting position, athletes hop to the 18-inch target on a single leg. After stabilizing, reach to starting position, then hop in the exact opposite direction back to starting position. Stabilize and reach to the target position.	4 (1 per direction)	5
5. Tuck Jump Progression Single tuck jump, soft landing	The athlete starts in athletic position with feet shoulder width apart. The athlete initiates a vertical jump with a single crouch downward while she extends her arms behind her. The athlete then swings her arms forward as she simultaneously jumps straight up and pulls her knees up as high as possible. At the peak of the jump, the athlete should be positioned in the air with thighs parallel to ground. The athlete should land softly, using a toe-to-midfoot rocker landing. The athlete should not continue this jump if she cannot control the high landing force or keep her knees aligned during landing. If she is unable to raise the knees to the proper height, instruct her to grasp the knees and then bring the thighs to horizontal.	10	2

Table 2
(continued)

Exercise Name	Description	Reps	Sets
6. Hamstring Strength Progression Flat double-legged pelvic bridge	The athlete lays supine with her hips and knees flexed and her feet planted on the ground. The athlete then extends her hips and elevates her trunk off of the ground to execute a pelvic bridge. This position should be held for 3 seconds before repeating the next repetition.	10	2
Phase 2 (Weeks 3–4)			
1. Single Leg Anterior Progression Jump–single-leg hold	The athlete begins the exercise in athletic position. She proceeds to jump forward, landing and balancing on 1 leg in a deep hold position.	8	2 (1 per side)
2. Single Leg Rotary Progression Single-leg 90-degree hold on soccer line	Perform the same hop hold as Phase 1 with the athlete's foot starting, rotating, and ending on a soccer line.	8	2 (1 per side)
3. Unanticipated Hop to Stabilization	Place 9 cones 18 inches apart. The coach will shout a sequence of 9 numbers from 1 to 9. Athletes can use any type of hop (anterior-posterior, medial-lateral, or a combination) to get to corresponding cones. Allow 3 seconds per hop.	9	3
4. Hop to Stabilization and Reach	From starting position, athletes hop to the 18-inch target on a single leg, hands on hips. After stabilizing, reach to starting position, then hop in the exact opposite direction back to starting position. Stabilize and reach to the target position while keeping hands on hips	4 (1 per direction)	5
5. Tuck Jump Progression Double tuck jump	Similar to the single tuck jump but with an additional jump performed immediately after the first. The athlete should focus on maintaining good form and minimizing time on the ground between jumps.	6	2
6. Hamstring Strength Progression Flat single-legged pelvic bridge	The athlete lays supine with her hips and knees flexed and a single foot planted on the ground and the contralateral leg fully extended. The athlete then extends her hip and trunk off the ground to execute a pelvic bridge. Hold this position for 3 seconds before repeating the next repetition.	10	2 (1 per side)

Table 2
(continued)

Exercise Name	Description	Reps	Sets
Phase 3 (Weeks 5–6)			
1. Single Leg Anterior Progression Hop-hold	Starting in a balanced position on 1 foot, the athlete hops forward, landing and balancing on one leg in a deep hold position.	8	2 (1 per side)
2. Single Leg Rotary Progression Single-leg 90-degree hold reaction ball catch on soccer line	Perform the same hop hold as Phase 1 with the athlete's foot starting, rotating, and ending on a soccer line. Upon landing, a ball will be passed back and forth with the athlete.	10	2 (1 per side)
3. Unanticipated Hop to Stabilization	Place 9 cones 18 inches apart. The coach will shout a sequence of 9 numbers from 1 to 9. Athletes can use any type of hop (anterior-posterior, medial-lateral, or a combination) to get to corresponding cones. Allow 1 second per hop.	9	3
4. Hop to Stabilization and Reach	From starting position, athletes hop to the 27-inch target on a single leg, hands on hips. After stabilizing, reach to starting position, then hop in the exact opposite direction back to starting position. Stabilize and reach to the target position. Athletes can use their arms to stabilize.	4 (1 per direction)	5
5. Tuck Jump Progression Repeated tuck jump	The athlete starts in the athletic position with her feet shoulder width apart. The athlete initiates a vertical jump with a single crouch downward while she extends her arms behind her. The athlete then swings her arms forward as she simultaneously jumps straight up and pulls her knees up as high as possible. At the peak of the jump the athlete should be positioned in the air with her thighs parallel to the ground. When landing, the athlete should immediately begin the next tuck jump.	10 seconds	2
6. Hamstring Strength Progression Flat single-legged pelvic bridge with ball	The athlete lays supine with her hips and knees flexed and a single foot planted on the ground. The athlete then extends her hip and trunk off the ground to execute a pelvic bridge. As she is extending her hips and elevating, she tosses the ball in the air and catches it. Hold this position for 3 seconds before repeating the next repetition.	10	2 (1 per side)

Table 2
(continued)

Exercise Name	Description	Reps	Sets
Phase 4 (Weeks 7–8)			
1. Single Leg Anterior Progression Hop-hold-hold	The athlete quickly hops forward twice, landing and balancing on one leg in a deep hold position.	8	2 (1 per side)
2. Single Leg Rotary Progression Single-leg 90-degree hold on soccer line with perturbations	The athlete completes the same exercise as phase 2, with a partner lightly perturbing a part of the athlete's body (shoulder, hip, waist).	8	2 (1 per side)
3. Unanticipated Hop to Stabilization	Place 9 cones 18 inches apart. The coach will shout a sequence of 9 numbers from 1 to 9. Athletes can use any type of hop (anterior-posterior, medial-lateral, or a combination) to get to corresponding cones. Allow 1 second per hop. If the athlete can do this error-free, she can do this sequence with closed eyes.	9	3
4. Hop to Stabilization and Reach	From starting position, athletes hop to the 27-inch target on a single leg, hands on hips. After stabilizing, reach to starting position, then hop in the exact opposite direction back to starting position. Stabilize and reach to the target position. Hands should be placed on hips while stabilizing.	4 (1 per direction)	5
5. Tuck Jump Progression Side-to-side tuck jumps	The athlete starts in the athletic position with her feet shoulder width apart. The athlete initiates a vertical jump over the soccer line with a single crouch downward while she extends her arms behind her. The athlete then swings her arms forward as she simultaneously jumps straight up and pulls her knees up as high as possible. At the peak of the jump the athlete should be positioned in the air with her thighs parallel to the ground. When landing, the athlete should immediately begin the next jump back to the other side of the line.	10 seconds	2

Table 2
(continued)

Exercise Name	Description	Reps	Sets
6. Hamstring Strength Progression Russian hamstring curl	The athlete kneels on the ground with her upper body straight, knees, and lower legs hip-width apart. Her arms are crossed. Have a partner pin her ankles firmly to the ground with both hands. The athlete slowly leans forward keeping upper body and hips straight. The straight body alignment should be maintained as long as possible. When this body position can no longer be maintained by the hamstrings, then use both hands to catch yourself. Use a push-up technique with arms to return to starting position.	10	2 (1 per side)
Phase 5 (Weeks 9–10)			
1. Single Leg Anterior Progression Crossover hop-hold-hold	The athlete quickly hops forward while alternating legs 3 times quickly, landing and balancing on one leg in a deep hold position.	8	2 (1 per side)
2. Single Leg Rotary Progression Single-leg 90 degree hold reaction ball on soccer line with perturbations	Exercises from phase 3 and phase 4 of this progression are combined.	8	2 (1 per side)
3. Unanticipated Hop to Stabilization	Place 9 cones 18 inches apart. The coach will shout a sequence of 9 numbers from 1 to 9. Athletes can use any type of hop (anterior-posterior, medial-lateral, or a combination) to get to corresponding cones. Allow 1 second per hop. If the athlete can do this error-free, she can do this sequence with closed eyes and hands on hips.	9	3
4. Hop to Stabilization and Reach	From starting position, athletes hop to the 36-inch target on a single leg, hands on hips. After stabilizing, reach to starting position, then hop in the exact opposite direction back to starting position. Stabilize and reach to the target position. Athletes can rely on arms for stabilization.	4 (1 per direction)	5

Table 2
(continued)

Exercise Name	Description	Reps	Sets
5. Tuck Jump Progression Side-to-side tuck jumps (same as phase 4)	The athlete starts in the athletic position with her feet shoulder width apart. The athlete initiates a vertical jump over the soccer line with a single crouch downward while she extends her arms behind her. The athlete then swings her arms forward as she simultaneously jumps straight up and pulls her knees up as high as possible. At the peak of the jump the athlete should be positioned in the air with her thighs parallel to the ground. When landing, the athlete should immediately begin the next jump back to the other side of the line.	10 seconds	2
6. Hamstring Strength Progression Russian hamstring curl (same as phase 4)	The athlete kneels on the ground with her upper body straight, knees, and lower legs hip-width apart. Her arms are crossed. Have a partner pin her ankles firmly to the ground with both hands. The athlete slowly leans forward keeping upper body and hips straight. The straight body alignment should be maintained as long as possible. When this body position can no longer be maintained by the hamstrings, then use both hands to catch yourself. Use a push-up technique with arms to return to starting position.	10	2 (1 per side)

Phase 5 (Weeks 9–10)

RESULTS

Athlete compliance for the IN group was noted weekly by individual coaches using attendance and exposure reports. Compliance was measured by dividing the total number of sessions attended by the total sessions offered. Compliance in the IN neuromuscular intervention was 95%.

For all athletes measured at preseason and postseason, there was a significant main effect of time on the tuck jump assessment score (P = .04). Both teams significantly reduced their TJA scores. The in-season trained group reduced their measured landing and jumping deficits from 5.4 ± 1.6 points to 4.9 ± 1.0 points following training and the season. In addition, athletes who performed standard soccer in-season training (CTRL) also showed a reduction from 5.8 ± 1.6 to 5.0 ± 1.5 points following a soccer season. There was not a significant interaction of training status (P = .65) between the IN and CTRL study groups.

DISCUSSION

Periodized strength and conditioning programs are quickly becoming the standard for high school sports. Due to the proposed positive effects of injury prevention training, this type of training should be included in a comprehensive program. Despite the demonstrated efficacy of injury prevention training for female athletes, compliance has historically been relatively low when the training is focused on injury prevention.[13] Combining injury prevention training with the team's regular preseason and in-season training may be the optimal way to increase compliance, as it merely alters the routine rather than making wholesale changes to their regimen. However, the current results do not support the use of in-season ACL intervention training to reduce measured TJA deficits above and beyond a standard in-season soccer protocol. There may be a uncovered dose-response relationship associated with neuromuscular training, which would improve the efficacy of this training protocol.[41] The inclusion of injury prevention training during the preseason may be a necessary component to achieve positive effects on risk factors associated with injury and may be an important limitation to the program presented in the current study.[42]

In addition, the importance of preseason training was further highlighted by the work of Ghilcrist and colleagues.[7] Based on these data, it appears that preseason training, the often-neglected training element, is responsible for the athletes' safety during the first half of the competitive season. By instituting a thorough preseason training regimen, the athletes could potentially see the benefits as soon as their competitive season begins. A positive dose-response relationship has been suggested in which 6 to 8 weeks of training is critical for inducing positive changes in injury prevention.[41,42] However, the volume of injury prevention training during the regular season may be too low to elicit desired effects, as a greater amount of time is dedicated to performance.

Further complicating the matter are the restrictions that most states have on contact time between players and coaches. The dates at which sports teams can begin practicing are set by each state to ensure student-athletes' safety, but these regulations also put a premium on the time when coaches are allowed to interact with their players. Sadly, injury prevention training often is first to get cut.[13] By combining injury prevention training with both the preseason and in-season training, the critical mass for improvements may be easier to achieve.

Vescovi and colleagues emphasized another key point in the rationale for the use of both preseason and in-season training. Their study showed that in-season injury prevention training alone was not sufficient to illicit any performance gains in a similar population.[43] This speaks to both the dose-response relationship and the need to incorporate performance goals for the training to improve compliance. Our TJA can be used as an injury prevention tool but also as a measurement of athletic performance.

Compliance

Compliance in any intervention is crucial. In this study, the compliance rate for the in-season intervention was 95%. Factors influencing such high compliance could include the motivational nature of this particular intervention, duration of the intervention, preseason versus in-season programs, athlete/trainer ratio, and type of instructor (coach or athletic trainer). Future research should attempt to tease out these differences. Bien[44] recently noted that increased compliance is more likely to occur in warm-up programs, rather than in interventions that do not precede an athletic practice. Results of a recent meta-analysis indicated a potential dose-response relationship between neuromuscular training compliance and reduction of ACL incidence rates.[41] High attendance and completion rates of prescribed neuromuscular training sessions appear to be an important component for preventing ACL injuries in young female athletes. Additions to the protocol aiming to increase athletic performance measures (eg, vertical jump, sprint speed, or strength) could improve compliance in future populations.

Response to Intervention

In a similar report, Brent and colleagues evaluated the effects of preseason-only and in-season neuromuscular training only to a standard soccer training season using the field-based evaluation used in the current study.[42] These authors reported that the preseason ACL intervention resulted in a 1.4-point (95% confidence interval, 0.6 to 2.2 points) reduction compared to this in-season neuromuscular or standard soccer training. In the current study, the IN group did not significantly reduce the number of mean flaws per video in comparison to control. Thus, the in-season neuromuscular intervention and regular soccer warm-ups have similar effects on TJA score, suggesting that participation in the sport itself could have some effect on tuck jump biomechanics (eg, a subject's progressive fitness level could translate into improved performance on the TJA). However, to achieve greater reductions in deficits, and potentially improve the efficacy of reduced injury risk at the onset of the competitive season, a preseason additive neuromuscular training protocol may be warranted.[7,16,42]

The time difference between the pre- and post-testing for IN and CTRL was only 5 weeks due to a relatively short soccer season. In a meta-analysis of studies with neuromuscular interventions, Hewett and coworkers concluded that for the program to be effective, it must have a minimum duration of 6 weeks,[21] while Bien concluded a minimum of 8 weeks was necessary for injury prevention.[44] Further studies should investigate whether starting an intervention earlier (in the preseason) and continuing it throughout the season, would lead to significant improvements compared to "typical" soccer training.

The tuck jump assessment allows a coach or clinician to evaluate an athlete's risk of injury without the use of expensive equipment. By using the TJA throughout the yearly training cycle, overall deficits can be targeted (**Fig. 2**) and progress can be monitored (**Fig. 1**), which may allow the neuromuscular training to be more thoroughly directed. Targeted training as suggested has been shown to improve the efficacy of similar training programs implemented during preseason and may benefit ACL injury prevention programs that are implemented during[45] the season as well. The results

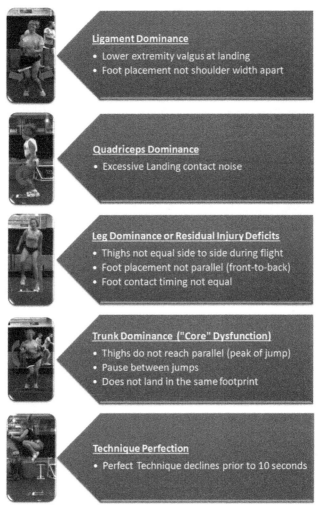

Fig. 2. Tuck jump assessment criteria grouped by modifiable risk factor categorizations. (*Reproduced from* Myer GD, Brent JL, Ford KR, Hewett TE. Real-time assessment and feedback techniques for use in neuromuscular training aimed to prevent ACL injury. Strength Conditioning J 2011;33(3):21-35; with permission.)

also indicate a potential dose-response to the neuromuscular training.[41,42] Preliminary results indicate that combining injury prevention training with the team's traditional sport training throughout the competitive season has added benefits in terms of reducing risk of ACL injury based on improvements to the athlete's TJA score. Future research is warranted to determine the relationship of reduced deficits gained from use of the presented techniques with actual reduction of injury in athletes treated with targeted training.

SUMMARY

Athletes measured pre- and post-training significantly decreased their mean total scores on the TJA after the intervention period and/or the season. However, subjects in the current study who received the in-season proprioceptive training did not reduce their deficits in the TJA above and beyond a standard soccer season training protocol. There may be a dose-response relationship to the neuromuscular training targeted to prevent ACL injury. Future research is warranted to determine if preseason combined with in-season maintenance training is optimal in improving biomechanics and reducing ACL injury risk. Both preseason and in-season neuromuscular training may be best used to help minimize the risk factors associated with ACL injuries, especially in the early season. Coaches can evaluate the training progress of their athletes using a field-based TJA with a significantly lower cost than previous methods.

REFERENCES

1. Mihata LC, Beutler AI, Boden BP. Comparing the incidence of anterior cruciate ligament injury in collegiate lacrosse, soccer, and basketball players: implications for anterior cruciate ligament mechanism and prevention. Am J Sports Med 2006;34(6): 899–904.
2. Agel J, Arendt EA, Bershadsky B. Anterior cruciate ligament injury in national collegiate athletic association basketball and soccer: a 13-year review. Am J Sports Med 2005;33(4):524–30.
3. Pappas E, Hagins M, Sheikhzadeh A, et al. Biomechanical differences between unilateral and bilateral landings from a jump: gender differences. Clin J Sport Med 2007;17(4):263–8.
4. Ford KR, Myer GD, Smith RL, et al. A comparison of dynamic coronal plane excursion between matched male and female athletes when performing single leg landings. Clin Biomech (Bristol, Avon) 2006;21(1):33–40.
5. Ford KR, Myer GD, Hewett TE. Valgus knee motion during landing in high school female and male basketball players. Med Sci Sports Exerc 2003;35(10):1745–50.
6. Kiani A, Hellquist E, Ahlqvist K, et al. Prevention of soccer-related knee injuries in teenaged girls. Arch Intern Med 2010;170(1):43–9.
7. Gilchrist J, Mandelbaum BR, Melancon H, et al. A randomized controlled trial to prevent noncontact anterior cruciate ligament injury in female collegiate soccer players. Am J Sports Med 2008;36(8):1476-83.
8. Steffen K, Myklebust G, Olsen OE, et al. Preventing injuries in female youth football: a cluster-randomized controlled trial. Scand J Med Sci Sports 2008;18(5):605--14.
9. Petersen W, Braun C, Bock W, et al. A controlled prospective case control study of a prevention training program in female team handball players: the German experience. Arch Orthop Trauma Surg 2006;125(9):614–21.
10. Pfeiffer RP, Shea KG, Roberts D, et al. Lack of effect of a knee ligament injury prevention program on the incidence of noncontact anterior cruciate ligament injury. J Bone Joint Surg Am 2006;88(8):1769–74.
11. Olsen OE, Myklebust G, Engebretsen L, et al. Exercises to prevent lower limb injuries in youth sports: cluster randomised controlled trial. BMJ 2005;330(7489):449.
12. Mandelbaum BR, Silvers HJ, Watanabe DS, et al. Effectiveness of a neuromuscular and proprioceptive training program in preventing anterior cruciate ligament injuries in female athletes: 2-year follow-up. Am J Sports Med 2005;33(7):1003–10.
13. Myklebust G, Engebretsen L, Braekken IH, et al. Prevention of anterior cruciate ligament injuries in female team handball players: a prospective intervention study over three seasons. Clin J Sport Med 2003;13(2):71–8.
14. Soderman K, Werner S, Pietila T, et al. Balance board training: prevention of traumatic injuries of the lower extremities in female soccer players? A prospective randomized intervention study. Knee Surg Sports Traumatol Arthrosc 2000;8(6):356–3.

15. Heidt RS Jr, Sweeterman LM, Carlonas RL, et al. Avoidance of soccer injuries with preseason conditioning. Am J Sports Med 2000;28(5):659–62.
16. Hewett TE, Lindenfeld TN, Riccobene JV, et al. The effect of neuromuscular training on the incidence of knee injury in female athletes. A prospective study. Am J Sports Med 1999;27(6):699–706.
17. Hewett TE, Myer GD, Ford KR. Reducing knee and anterior cruciate ligament injuries among female athletes: a systematic review of neuromuscular training interventions. J Knee Surg 2005;18(1):82–8.
18. Hewett TE, Ford KR, Myer GD. Anterior cruciate ligament injuries in female athletes: Part 2, a meta-analysis of neuromuscular interventions aimed at injury prevention. Am J Sports Med 2006;34(3):490–8.
19. Pollard CD, Sigward SM, Ota S, et al. The influence of in-season injury prevention training on lower-extremity kinematics during landing in female soccer players. Clin J Sport Med 2006;16(3):223–7.
20. Zebis MK, Bencke J, Andersen LL, et al. The effects of neuromuscular training on knee joint motor control during sidecutting in female elite soccer and handball players. Clin J Sport Med 2008;18(4):329–37.
21. Hewett TE, Myer GD, Ford KR, et al. Biomechanical measures of neuromuscular control and valgus loading of the knee predict anterior cruciate ligament injury risk in female athletes: a prospective study. Am J Sports Med 2005;33(4):492–501.
22. Padua DA, Marshall SW, Beutler AI, et al. Prospective cohort study of biomechanical risk factors of ACL injury: the JUMP-ACL Study. Presented at the American Orthopaedic Society of Sports Medicine Annual Meeting. Keystone, CO, 2009. p. 393-5.
23. Hewett TE, Ford KR, Myer GD, et al. Gender differences in hip adduction motion and torque during a single leg agility maneuver. J Orthop Res 2006;24(3):416–21.
24. Kernozek TW, Torry MR, et al. Gender differences in frontal and sagittal plane biomechanics during drop landings. Med Sci Sports Exerc 2005;37(6):1003–12 [discussion: 1013].
25. Hewett TE, Myer GD, Ford KR. Decrease in neuromuscular control about the knee with maturation in female athletes. J Bone Joint Surg Am 2004;86-A(8):1601–8.
26. McLean SG, Huang X, Su A, et al. Sagittal plane biomechanics cannot injure the ACL during sidestep cutting. Clin Biomech (Bristol, Avon) 2004;19:828–38.
27. Zeller BL, McCrory JL, Kibler WB, et al. Differences in kinematics and electromyographic activity between men and women during the single-legged squat. Am J Sport Med 2003;31(3):449–56.
28. Chappell JD, Yu B, Kirkendall DT, et al. A comparison of knee kinetics between male and female recreational athletes in stop-jump tasks. Am J Sports Med 2002;30(2):261–7.
29. Malinzak RA, Colby SM, Kirkendall DT, et al. A comparison of knee joint motion patterns between men and women in selected athletic tasks. Clin Biomech (Bristol, Avon) 2001;16(5):438–45.
30. Krosshaug T, Nakamae A, Boden BP, et al. Mechanisms of anterior cruciate ligament injury in basketball: video analysis of 39 cases. Am J Sports Med 2007;35(3):359–67.
31. Olsen OE, Myklebust G, Engebretsen L, et al. Injury mechanisms for anterior cruciate ligament injuries in team handball: a systematic video analysis. Am J Sports Med 2004;32(4):1002–12.
32. Boden BP, Dean GS, Feagin JA, et al. Mechanisms of anterior cruciate ligament injury. Orthopedics 2000;23(6):573–8.
33. Myer GD, Ford KR, Hewett TE. New method to identify athletes at high risk of ACL injury using clinic-based measurements and freeware computer analysis. Br J Sports Med 2011;45(4):238–44.

34. Myer GD, Ford KR, Khoury J, et al. Three-dimensional motion analysis validation of a clinic-based nomogram designed to identify high ACL injury risk in female athletes. Physician Sports Med 2011;39(1):19–28.

35. Myer GD, Ford KR, Khoury J, et al. Development and validation of a clinic-based prediction tool to identify female athletes at high risk for anterior cruciate ligament injury. Am J Sports Med 2010;38(10):2025–33.

36. Myer GD, Brent JL, Ford KR, et al. Real-time assessment and feedback techniques for use in neuromuscular training aimed to prevent ACL injury. Strength Cond J 2011;33(3):21–35.

37. Myer GD, Ford KR, Hewett TE. Tuck jump assessment for reducing anterior cruciate ligament injury risk. Athl Ther Today 2008;13(5):39–44.

38. Myer GD, Brent JL, Ford KR, et al. A pilot study to determine the effect of trunk and hip focused neuromuscular training on hip and knee isokinetic strength. Br J Sports Med 2008;42(7):614–9.

39. Myer GD, Chu DA, Brent JL, et al. Trunk and hip control neuromuscular training for the prevention of knee joint injury. Clin Sports Med 2008;27(3):425–48, ix.

40. Hewett TE, Stroupe AL, Nance TA, et al. Plyometric training in female athletes. Decreased impact forces and increased hamstring torques. Am J Sports Med 1996;24(6):765–73.

41. Sugimoto D, Myer GD, Bush HM, et al. The effects of compliance with neuromuscular training on anterior cruciate ligament injury risk reduction in young female athletes: a meta-analysis. Presented at the National Athletic Training Association Annual Meeting. New Orleans, LA, 2011.

42. Brent JL, Klugman MA, Myer GD, et al. The effects of preseason and in-season neuromuscular training on the tuck jump assessment: a test used to identify risk of ACL injury in female athletes. National Strength and Conditioning Association Annual Meeting. 2010.

43. Vescovi JD, VanHeest JL. Effects of an anterior cruciate ligament injury prevention program on performance in adolescent female soccer players. Scand J Med Sci Sports 2010;20(3):394–402.

44. Bien DP. Rationale and implementation of anterior cruciate ligament injury prevention warm-up programs in female athletes. J Strength Cond Res 2011;25(1):271–85.

45. Myer GD, Ford KR, Brent JL, et al. Differential neuromuscular training effects on ACL injury risk factors in "high-risk" versus "low-risk" athletes. BMC Musculoskelet Disord 2007;8(39):1–7.

Stopping Sports Injuries in Young Athletes

Destin E. Hill, MD*, James R. Andrews, MD

KEYWORDS

• Pediatric • Sports • Injuries • Overuse • Prevention
• Athlete

The number of children playing recreational sports increases every year.[1] Over 30 million children play organized sports in the United States yearly.[1] Additionally, it is estimated that over 7.6 million high school students participated in high school sports in 2009–2010.[2] This number does not include those young athletes that participated in club sports, all-star teams, or recreational leagues that are not affiliated with their local school. High school athletes account for more than 2 million injuries annually, including over 500,000 physician visits and 30,000 hospitalizations.[3,4] More than 3.5 million children under the age of 14 are seen annually for sports-related injuries.[1] While these numbers are staggering, they continue to rise yearly.

In addition to the steadily rising rate of young athletes in the United States, the prevalence of "sport specialization" is also becoming increasingly popular. The days of the multisport athlete are rapidly fading. Kids today are focusing on one sport beginning at an early age. These young, one-sport athletes are typically participating in year-round competition with nonexistent rest periods between the seasons. By the time many of these athletes reach high school, they are competing on multiple teams with overlapping seasons and virtually no time off. Complicating the issue with many of these young athletes is their immature bones, poor biomechanics, a lack of knowledgeable coaching, and inadequate conditioning. All of these factors combined quickly lead to a recipe for injury.

The emergence of the "one-sport athlete" has also predictably led to a disturbing rise in overuse injuries. Instead of allowing an athlete to rest a particular body part (i.e. pitching arm) by participating in other sports during the year, the one-sport athlete continuously uses the same body parts year round. The nonstop use of the same body parts has led to an increase in overuse injuries of these body parts. It is now estimated that over 50% of all injuries in middle and high school athletes are from overuse.[1] Previous generations of athletes were given months of rest simply by playing other sports. Today, the one-sport athletes are pushed to perform at an

The authors have nothing to disclose.
American Sports Medicine Institute, 2660 10th Avenue South, Suite 505, Birmingham, AL 35205, USA
* Corresponding author.
E-mail address: destinhill@gmail.com

Clin Sports Med 30 (2011) 841–849
doi:10.1016/j.csm.2011.07.003   sportsmed.theclinics.com

exceptionally high level for extended periods without sufficient rest to allow their bodies to recover. The senior author who has studied this rise in overuse injuries, Dr James R. Andrews, has recommended that young athletes take several months away from their sport each year in order to allow their body to recuperate from the grueling sports seasons.

One example of this epidemic of overuse injuries is exemplified by the 5- to 7-fold increase in shoulder and elbow injuries since 2000 in youth baseball players.[5] Injuries that were once exclusively diagnosed in the professional pitcher are now being seen in adolescent pitchers. It was previously unheard of for a teenage baseball player to tear the ulnar collateral ligament (Tommy John ligament), but today, it is quite common for a high school baseball team to have at least one player that has undergone ulnar collateral ligament reconstruction surgery. The truly frightening aspect of this injury trend is that it continues to escalate every year. Our young athletes' health is on a runaway train and something needs to be done to stop it.

HISTORY

In 2007, the alarming escalation in overuse injuries in young athletes caught the attention of the American Orthopaedic Society for Sports Medicine (AOSSM). Members of the AOSSM's Board of Directors, initiated by Dr Andrews, decided that the issue of overuse injuries was becoming critical and it needed to be addressed. In response to the significant rise in youth sports injuries, the STOP (Sports Trauma and Overuse Prevention) Sports Injuries campaign was created in 2007. After the campaign was formed, a steering committee was then selected to investigate what types of activities and materials needed to be developed to combat the problem. In late 2009, the planning and fundraising efforts began in earnest, along with support from organizational partners including the American Academy of Orthopaedic Surgeons (AAOS), the American Academy of Pediatrics (AAP), the National Athletic Trainers' Association (NATA), the American Medical Society for Sports Medicine (AMSSM), the Sports Physical Therapy Section of the American Physical Therapy Association, and SAFE Kids USA. These organizations shared AOSSM's concern about the drastic increase in youth sports injuries and partnered together under the common goal of the STOP Sports Injuries movement. Since its inception in 2007, STOP Sports Injuries has worked tirelessly to decrease the overuse injuries in young athletes.

PURPOSE

STOP Sports Injuries mission statement of "keeping kids in the game for life" serves as the compass for the movement. The campaign not only concentrates on injury reduction but also highlights how playing safe and aware can increase a child's athletic career, improve teamwork, reduce obesity rates, and create a life-long love of exercise and healthy activity. The program's goal is to achieve a nationwide impact through a variety of media outlets as well as corporate and individual partnerships. The STOP Sports Injuries program has not only recognized an epidemic occurring in our young athletes but has also set out to reverse the trend through a wide array of public service announcements, conferences, presentations, and an interactive website.

EDUCATIONAL INITIATIVE

As stated, the STOP Sports Injuries educational initiative has worked diligently to educate athletes, their parents, coaches, and health care professionals about the danger of overuse injuries. This includes public service announcements, posters, DVDs, brochures, electronic newsletters, an interactive website, and even social media sites like Facebook and Twitter. The comprehensive public outreach program focuses on the importance of sports safety, specifically relating to overuse and trauma injuries. However, local, grassroots outreach will continue to be the key to the campaign's success.

The establishment of pitch counts in youth baseball is just one example of the educational initiatives of the STOP campaign. Pitch counts have become a hot topic in youth baseball circles over the last several years. In years past, youth pitchers threw without limitations. Some youth baseball organizations had a maximum number of innings pitched per game/week; however, this is an exceptionally inaccurate way to monitor a young pitcher's workload. For example, a particular adolescent pitcher could throw 10 pitches in one inning and 50 pitches the next inning. Even though the young pitcher technically threw only 2 innings, the workload on that pitcher's arm during those 2 innings was drastically different. Additionally, during one game a pitcher may throw 60 pitches and the next game 120 pitches, yet stay under the innings limit during each game. The innings count, because it does not accurately measure the workload on a young pitcher's arm, does not serve to protect the athlete's arm.

In addition to a lack of pitch counts, there were also no guidelines on the number of days of rest a particular player needed after pitching. Most major league pitchers today are given 4 to 5 days of complete rest before pitching again, yet the same could not be said of our adolescent pitchers. Most competitive youth baseball teams use their 1 or 2 best pitchers for every game, including weekend-long tournaments. Teams can play upward of half a dozen games in these weekend tournaments with the teams' best pitchers throwing multiple times throughout. The result of no guidelines on days of rest after pitching has led to the overuse of a team's best pitchers. Additionally, the drive to win has allowed coaches, players, and parents to tolerate the overuse of their young pitchers. Not surprisingly, a 5- to 7-fold increase in elbow and shoulder injuries has been documented in young pitchers since 2000.[5]

The lack of pitch counts and guidelines for rest days after pitching led the STOP Sports Injuries campaign to unconditionally support pitch count limits and endorse adequate days of rest after pitching, as first addressed and recommended by USA Baseball, the official organization of amateur baseball in the United States, in 2006. In 2007, Little League Baseball became the first youth baseball organization to officially adopt a pitch count.[6] Countless youth baseball organizations have followed Little League's groundbreaking initiative over the next few years. The purpose of the pitch count limits and rest day requirements is to protect the young pitcher from overuse injuries. Too many young pitchers are developing injuries that are entirely preventable with some education. Despite the significant progress that has been made in youth baseball, there are still many youth baseball organizations across the country that have not adopted pitch count or rest day guidelines. The STOP campaign will continue to work vigorously with these organizations to encourage pitch counts and mandate days of rest after pitching.

The critical issue of pitch counts led Dr Glenn Fleisig, research director of The American Sports Medicine Institute (ASMI) in Birmingham, Alabama, and Dr Andrews, as its medical director, to develop a position statement in 2009 on pitch counts for young pitchers. They used years of data collected at ASMI to establish recommendations on pitch count limits for pitchers of all ages (**Table 1**). They also created a recommendation on days of rest required after pitching based on the number of pitches thrown and the age of the athlete (**Table 2**). Furthermore, Drs Fleisig and

Table 1	
Pitch counts by age	
Age (yr)	**Number of Pitches**
17–18	105
13–16	95
11–12	85
9–10	75
7–8	50

Andrews developed a recommendation on the appropriate age for a young pitcher to begin learning various pitches (**Table 3**). These recommendations were first adopted by USA Baseball and have since been embraced by the STOP Sports Injuries initiative.

In addition to continually educating the American public on the importance of pitch counts, the STOP Sports Injuries movement is also working to combat concussions, heat illness, improper tackling techniques in football, and many other injuries common in young athletes. The STOP Sports Injuries campaign desires to protect young athletes in many sports from preventable injuries. The campaign focuses on approximately 20 primary sports that were thought to be essential in decreasing the prevalence of overuse injuries (**Box 1**). These primary sports are not only some of the most popular sports in America, but they also provide an opportunity to drastically improve injury rates among the participants.

FUNDING

Financial support for the STOP Sport Injuries operation comes from a multitude of sources. The campaign is supported by health organizations such as the AAP, the National Strength and Conditioning Association (NSCA), NATA, and the Professional Baseball Athletic Trainers Association among many others. Along with numerous private practice sports medicine groups, several cutting-edge medical institutions and hospitals across the country have joined the STOP Sports Injuries team. Corporate sponsorship partners such as DePuy, Arthrex, and Smith & Nephew assist in furthering the spread of STOP's message as well. Even individuals and sports teams can join the movement by donating to the campaign. The STOP website provides more information on how corporations, medical groups, and individuals can help support the message.

RESOURCES

The STOP Sports Injuries website (www.stopsportsinjuries.org) has a tremendous amount of educational information for all interest levels.[7] Whether the individual is a

Table 2		
Rest periods required by age for pitches thrown		
Ages 7–16	**Ages 17–18**	**Days of Rest**
61+ pitches	76+ pitches	3
41–60 pitches	51–75 pitches	2
21–40 pitches	26–50 pitches	1
1–20 pitches	1–25 pitches	None

Table 3 Age recommendations for learning particular pitches	
Pitch	Age (yr)
Fastball	8 ± 2
Slider	16 ± 2
Change-up	10 ± 3
Forkball	16 ± 2
Curveball	14 ± 2
Knuckleball	15 ± 3
Screwball	17 ± 2

coach, parent, athlete, or health care provider, the website has information geared toward them. It serves as the epicenter for the movement by providing groundbreaking medical research on a user-friendly website.

For the coaches of young athletes, the website contains information to assist them in teaching their athletes how to safely participate in sports through practice tips, nutrition advice, and competition guidelines. It also gives the coach some practical help on how to deal with difficult and demanding parents. There are also injury prevention tips listed by sport directly on the website. These tips can be incorporated by the coach into their team's warm-ups, practices, and/or competitions to decrease the risk of injuries. Additionally, the website contains free posters and other educational information that can be printed and placed in a locker room, gym, or dugout to raise awareness for safe sports participation.

The STOP website not only provides information for coaches but also has resources for the parents of young athletes. Most parents are markedly unaware of injury risk factors and therefore underestimate these risk factors and subsequent injury rates associated with a specific sport. The resources for parents include advice on common injury risk factors, common injuries for each sport, injury prevention techniques, and even when to have their child evaluated by a medical professional for

Box 1 STOP Sports Injuries primary sports	
Baseball	Martial arts
Basketball	Rowing
Cheerleading	Rugby
Dance	Running
Field hockey	Skiing and snowboarding
Figure skating	Soccer
Football	Softball
Golf	Swimming
Gymnastics	Tennis
Hockey	Volleyball
Lacrosse	Wrestling

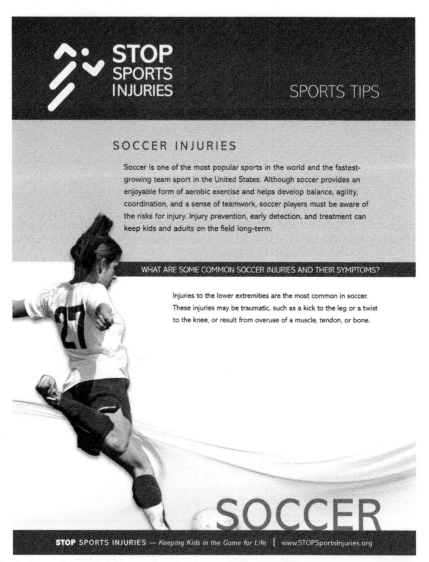

Fig. 1. Example of injury prevention tips for a specific sport (soccer). (*From* the STOP Sports Injuries website: http://www.stopsportsinjuries.org/soccer-injury-prevention.aspx; with permission from the American Orthopaedic Society for Sports Medicine. All rights reserved.)

a possible injury. If a parent wants to know how to treat a wrist or ankle sprain for their cheerleader or basketball player, he or she can check out the "Parents Resources" section. The website also serves to educate parents regarding youth baseball pitch counts (see **Table 1**) and when to allow your child to begin throwing a curveball, slider, or knuckleball (see **Table 3**). There are also medical consensus statements on athletic participation in athletes with sickle cell trait and other various medical conditions. Another aspect of the STOP Sports Injuries website that all parents should become familiar with is the educational material on concussions and heat illness. These resources can help parents recognize common symptoms of a concussion or

WHAT ARE SOME COMMON SOCCER INJURIES?

Lower Extremity Injuries
Sprains and strains are the most common lower extremity injuries. The severity of these injuries varies. Cartilage tears and anterior cruciate ligament (ACL) sprains in the knee are some of the more common injuries that may require surgery. Other injuries include fractures and contusions from direct blows to the body.

Overuse Lower Extremity Injuries
Shin splints (soreness in the calf), patellar tendinitis (pain in the knee), and Achilles tendinitis (pain in the back of the ankle) are some of the more common soccer overuse conditions. Soccer players are also prone to groin pulls and thigh and calf muscle strains.

Stress fractures occur when the bone becomes weak from overuse. It is often difficult to distinguish stress fractures from soft tissue injury. If pain develops in any part of your lower extremity and does not clearly improve after a few days of rest, a physician should be consulted to determine whether a stress fracture is present.

Upper Extremity Injuries
Injuries to the upper extremities usually occur from falling on an outstretched arm or from player-to-player contact. These conditions include wrist sprains, wrist fractures, and shoulder dislocations.

Head, Neck, and Face Injuries
Injuries to the head, neck, and face include cuts and bruises, fractures, neck sprains, and concussions. A concussion is any alteration in an athlete's mental state due to head trauma and should always be evaluated by a physician. Not all those who experience a concussion lose consciousness.

HOW ARE SOCCER INJURIES TREATED?

Participation should be stopped immediately until any injury is evaluated and treated properly. Most injuries are minor and can be treated by a short period of rest, ice, and elevation. If a trained health care professional such as a sports medicine physician or athletic trainer is available to evaluate an injury, often a decision can be made to allow an athlete to continue playing immediately. The athlete should return to play only when clearance is granted by a health care professional.

Overuse injuries can be treated with a short period of rest, which means that the athlete can continue to perform or practice some activities with modifications. In many cases, pushing through pain can be harmful,

especially for stress fractures, knee ligament injuries, and any injury to the head or neck. Contact your doctor for proper diagnosis and treatment of any injury that does not improve after a few days of rest.

You should return to play only when clearance is granted by a health care professional.

HOW CAN SOCCER INJURIES BE PREVENTED?

- Have a pre-season physical examination and follow your doctor's recommendations
- Use well-fitting cleats and shin guards — there is some evidence that molded and multi-studded cleats are safer than screw-in cleats
- Be aware of poor field conditions that can increase injury rates
- Use properly sized synthetic balls — leather balls that can become waterlogged and heavy are more dangerous, especially when heading
- Watch out for mobile goals that can fall on players and request fixed goals whenever possible
- Hydrate adequately — waiting until you are thirsty is often too late to hydrate properly
- Pay attention to environmental recommendations, especially in relation to excessively hot and humid weather, to help avoid heat illness
- Maintain proper fitness — injury rates are higher in athletes who have not adequately prepared physically.
- After a period of inactivity, progress gradually back to full-contact soccer through activities such as aerobic conditioning, strength training, and agility training.
- Avoid overuse injuries — more is not always better! Many sports medicine specialists believe that it is beneficial to take at least one season off each year. Try to avoid the pressure that is now exerted on many young athletes to over-train. Listen to your body and decrease training time and intensity if pain or discomfort develops. This will reduce the risk of injury and help avoid "burn-out"
- Speak with a sports medicine professional or athletic trainer if you have any concerns about injuries or prevention strategies

EXPERT CONSULTANTS

Rob Burger, MD
Kenneth Fine, MD

Sports Tips provide general information only and are not a substitute for your own good judgement or consultation with a physician. To order multiple copies of this fact sheet or learn more about sports injury prevention, please visit www.STOPSportsInjuries.org.

STOP SPORTS INJURIES

STOP SPORTS INJURIES — Keeping Kids in the Game for Life | www.STOPSportsInjuries.org

Fig. 1. (*continued*)

heat illness. It also gives parents instructions on what to do if their child is exhibiting any symptoms of these conditions.

Athletes can also be directed to the STOP Sports Injuries website. They can find injury prevention tips created specifically for their sport, whether they participate in soccer, golf, football, snowboarding, dancing, or any sport in between (**Fig. 1**). The athletes can also find practice and performance strategies that can help them safely maximize their athletic ability. Additionally, there is information that educates the athlete on when they should let their parents or coach know about a possible injury.

In addition to information for coaches, parents, and athletes, the STOP Sports Injuries website has resources for the sports medicine health care provider. It contains medical consensus statements on concussions, heat illness, and athletes with HIV. There are also guidelines that discuss return to play for the injured athlete and helpful instructions for the management of a mass participation event. The website even has a PowerPoint presentation that can be downloaded and used for educational purposes in the local community to help educate others on preventing sports injuries.

The STOP Sports Injuries website contains information geared toward any individual interested in sports. A blog written by nationally recognized healthcare experts

Box 2	
STOP Sports Injuries Council of Champions	
James R. Andrews, MD *Co-Chair*	**James Justice** Owner, Greenbriar Resort
Neal ElAttrache, MD *Co-Chair*	**Stephen Keener** *President & CEO, Little League International*
Hank Aaron *Hall of Fame Baseball Player/Atlanta Braves*	**Ian Lawson** *President, DePuy Mitek*
Marjorie Albohm *President, NATA*	**Dennis Lewin** *Chairman, Board of Directors, Little League Baseball International*
Bonnie Blair *Speed Skating Olympic Champion*	**Howie Long** *Former NFL Player, NFL Sportscaster, Fox Network*
Nicholas Bolletieri *World Champion Tennis Coach*	**Renaldo Nehimiah** *Director, Track & Field Worldwide*
Sam Bradford *2008 Heisman Trophy Winner*	**Teri McCambridge, MD** *Chairperson, AAP Council on Sports Medicine & Fitness*
Dale Brown *Dale Brown Enterprises*	**Renaldo Nehimiah** *Former Track and Field Record Holder*
John Callaghan, MD *President, AAOS*	**Jack Nicklaus** *Golden Bear Enterprises/Professional Golfer*
Chaplain Richard Camp, Jr. *Former Nationally Ranked Track & Field Athlete*	**Jerry Pate** Former, Professional Golfer
Tom Condon Football Agent	**Rick Peterson** *Milwaukee Brewers Pitching Coach*
Delos Cosgrove, MD *CEO, Cleveland Clinic*	**Christie Rampone** *WNT U.S. Soccer*
Joe Gibbs *Founder, Golf Channel*	**John Smoltz** *MLB Pitcher*
Eric Heiden, MD *Olympic Speed Skater and Orthopaedic Surgeon*	**Bart Starr** *Former Green Bay Packer Quarterback*
Jay R. Hoffman *President, NSCA*	**Mitchell Stoller** *President and CEO, SAFE Kids Worldwide*
Bo Jackson *Professional Multi-Sport Athlete*	**Jim Wilson** *Chairman, Jim Wilson & Assoc*

From the STOP Sports Injuries website: http://www.stopsportsinjuries.org/soccer-injury-prevention. aspx; with permission from the American Orthopaedic Society for Sports Medicine. All rights reserved.

discusses a wide variety of topics including warming up, stretching, and exercising in the cold, among many others. Podcasts discussing current issues in sports medicine are also available for downloading to a computer. The website also contains videos of news reports and interviews on topics such as baseball pitch counts and how to keep athletes properly hydrated. There are even cameo appearances by former Atlanta Braves pitcher John Smoltz and current St Louis Rams quarterback Sam Bradford (both Smoltz and Bradford are members of STOP Sports Injuries Council of Champions; **Box 2** shows a complete list of the STOP Sports Injuries Council of Champions).

The website is not the only way to keep up to date with the STOP Sports Injuries campaign. They can also be found on social media sites like Facebook and Twitter (@SportsSafety).

SUMMARY

The alarming rise in youth sports injuries in the United States is an epidemic that the STOP Sports Injuries campaign is working diligently to combat. Through educational initiatives directed at coaches, parents, athletes, and health care professionals, the disturbing trend can be reversed. One objective of the STOP Sports Injuries campaign is to "keep kids on the playing field and out of the operating room." This goal can be realized with continued education. In fact, significant progress has already been realized in several sports, as exemplified by the development of pitch count limits in many of the youth baseball organizations across the country. Nevertheless, there is still plenty of work to be done in protecting our young athletes from overuse injuries. With the help of countless corporate sponsors, medical institutions, medical societies, health care professionals, parents, coaches, and athletes, we can all make a difference in protecting our young athletes from preventable overuse injuries. Let's all work together to stop sports injuries . . . and keep kids in the game for life.

ACKNOWLEDGMENTS

The authors would like to thank Glenn Dortch of ASMI for his wisdom and assistance during the writing of this article.

REFERENCES

1. Safe Kids USA Campaign. Available at: http://www.safekids.org/our-work/research/fact-sheets/sport-and-recreation-safety-fact-sheet.html. Accessed December 11, 2010.
2. National Federation of State High School Associations. Available at: http://www.nfhs.org/content.aspx?id=3282. Accessed January 14, 2011.
3. Powell J, Barber-Foss K. Injury patterns in selected high school sports: a review of the 1995–1997 seasons. J Athl Train 1999;34:277–84.
4. Center for Disease Control and Prevention. Available at: http://www.cdc.gov/safechild/Sports_Injuries/index.html. Accessed December 15, 2010.
5. Andrews J, Fleisig G. Protecting Young Pitching Arms: The Little League Pitch Count Regulation Guide for Parents, Coaches, and League Officials. Little League Baseball 2008. Available at: http://www.littleleague.org/Assets/old_assets/media/pitch_count_publication_2008.pdf. Accessed January 6, 2011.
6. Dick P. Pitch count, not innings, to limit Little Leaguer hurlers. Available at: http://www.usatoday.com/sports/baseball/llws/2006-08-27-little-league-pitch-count_x.htm. Accessed January 14, 2011.
7. STOP Sports Injuries. Available at: http://www.stopsportsinjuries.org/. Accessed November 7, 2010.

Index

Note: Page numbers of article titles are in **boldface** type.

doi:10.1016/S0278-5919(11)00091-3
0278-5919/11/$ – see front matter © 2011 Elsevier Inc. All rights reserved.
sportsmed.theclinics.com

United States Postal Service

Statement of Ownership, Management, and Circulation
(All Periodicals Publications Except Requestor Publications)

1. Publication Title	2. Publication Number									3. Filing Date
Clinics in Sports Medicine	0	0	0	-	7	0	0	2		9/16/11

4. Issue Frequency	5. Number of Issues Published Annually	6. Annual Subscription Price
Jan, Apr, Jul, Oct	4	$297.00

7. Complete Mailing Address of Known Office of Publication (Not printer) (Street, city, county, state, and ZIP+4®)

Elsevier Inc.
360 Park Avenue South
New York, NY 10010-1710

Contact Person
Stephen Bushing

Telephone (Include area code)
215-239-3688

8. Complete Mailing Address of Headquarters or General Business Office of Publisher (Not printer)

Elsevier Inc., 360 Park Avenue South, New York, NY 10010-1710

9. Full Names and Complete Mailing Addresses of Publisher, Editor, and Managing Editor (Do not leave blank)

Publisher (Name and complete mailing address)

Kim Murphy, Elsevier, Inc., 1600 John F. Kennedy Blvd. Suite 1800, Philadelphia, PA 19103-2899

Editor (Name and complete mailing address)

Jessica McCool, Elsevier, Inc., 1600 John F. Kennedy Blvd. Suite 1800, Philadelphia, PA 19103-2899

Managing Editor (Name and complete mailing address)

Barbara Cohen-Kligerman, Elsevier, Inc., 1600 John F. Kennedy Blvd. Suite 1800, Philadelphia, PA 19103-2899

10. Owner (Do not leave blank. If the publication is owned by a corporation, give the name and address of the corporation immediately followed by the names and addresses of all stockholders owning or holding 1 percent or more of the total amount of stock. If not owned by a corporation, give the names and addresses of the individual owners. If owned by a partnership or other unincorporated firm, give its name and address as well as those of each individual owner. If the publication is published by a nonprofit organization, give its name and address.)

Full Name	Complete Mailing Address
Wholly owned subsidiary of	4520 East-West Highway
Reed/Elsevier, US holdings	Bethesda, MD 20814

11. Known Bondholders, Mortgagees, and Other Security Holders Owning or Holding 1 Percent or More of Total Amount of Bonds, Mortgages, or Other Securities. If none, check box ☐ None

Full Name	Complete Mailing Address
N/A	

12. Tax Status (For completion by nonprofit organizations authorized to mail at nonprofit rates) (Check one)
The purpose, function, and nonprofit status of this organization and the exempt status for federal income tax purposes:
☐ Has Not Changed During Preceding 12 Months
☐ Has Changed During Preceding 12 Months (Publisher must submit explanation of change with this statement)

PS Form 3526, September 2007 (Page 1 of 3 (Instructions Page 3)) PSN 7530-01-000-9931 PRIVACY NOTICE: See our Privacy policy in www.usps.com

---

13. Publication Title	14. Issue Date for Circulation Data Below
Clinics in Sports Medicine	July 2011

15. Extent and Nature of Circulation				Average No. Copies Each Issue During Preceding 12 Months	No. Copies of Single Issue Published Nearest to Filing Date
a. Total Number of Copies (Net press run)				1306	1250
b. Paid Circulation (By Mail and Outside the Mail)	(1)	Mailed Outside-County Paid Subscriptions Stated on PS Form 3541 (Include paid distribution above nominal rate, advertiser's proof copies, and exchange copies)		700	640
	(2)	Mailed In-County Paid Subscriptions Stated on PS Form 3541 (Include paid distribution above nominal rate, advertiser's proof copies, and exchange copies)			
	(3)	Paid Distribution Outside the Mails Including Sales Through Dealers and Carriers, Street Vendors, Counter Sales, and Other Paid Distribution Outside USPS®		133	125
	(4)	Paid Distribution by Other Classes Mailed Through the USPS (e.g. First-Class Mail®)			
c. Total Paid Distribution (Sum of 15b (1), (2), (3), and (4))			▲	833	765
d. Free or Nominal Rate Distribution (By Mail and Outside the Mail)	(1)	Free or Nominal Rate Outside-County Copies Included on PS Form 3541		54	63
	(2)	Free or Nominal Rate In-County Copies Included on PS Form 3541			
	(3)	Free or Nominal Rate Copies Mailed at Other Classes Through the USPS (e.g. First-Class Mail)			
	(4)	Free or Nominal Rate Distribution Outside the Mail (Carriers or other means)			
e. Total Free or Nominal Rate Distribution (Sum of 15d (1), (2), (3) and (4))			▲	54	63
f. Total Distribution (Sum of 15c and 15e)			▲	887	828
g. Copies not Distributed (See instructions to publishers #4 (page #3))			▲	419	422
h. Total (Sum of 15f and g)			▲	1306	1250
i. Percent Paid (15c divided by 15f times 100)				93.91%	92.39%

16. Publication of Statement of Ownership
☐ If the publication is a general publication, publication of this statement is required. Will be printed ☐ Publication not required
in the October 2011 issue of this publication.

17. Signature and Title of Editor, Publisher, Business Manager, or Owner	Date
Stephen R. Bushing	September 16, 2011
Stephen R. Bushing – Inventory/Distribution Coordinator	

I certify that all information furnished on this form is true and complete. I understand that anyone who furnishes false or misleading information on this form or who omits material or information requested on the form may be subject to criminal sanctions (including fines and imprisonment) and/or civil sanctions (including civil penalties).

PS Form 3526, September 2007 (Page 2 of 3)

Moving?

Make sure your subscription moves with you!

To notify us of your new address, find your **Clinics Account Number** (located on your mailing label above your name), and contact customer service at:

Email: journalscustomerservice-usa@elsevier.com

800-654-2452 (subscribers in the U.S. & Canada)
314-447-8871 (subscribers outside of the U.S. & Canada)

Fax number: 314-447-8029

Elsevier Health Sciences Division
Subscription Customer Service
3251 Riverport Lane
Maryland Heights, MO 63043

Printed and bound by CPI Group (UK) Ltd, Croydon, CR0 4YY

03/10/2024

01040458-0017